Maryon Stewart's Zest For Life Plan

Maryon Stewart studied preventive dentistry and nutrition at the Royal Dental Hospital in London and worked as a counsellor with nutritional doctors in England for four years. At the beginning of 1984 she set up the PMT Advisory Service which has subsequently helped thousands of women worldwide. In 1987 she launched the Women's Nutritional Advisory Service which now provides broader help to women of all ages.

Maryon Stewart is the author of the bestselling books *Beat the Menopause Without HRT*, *No More PMS*, now in its third edition, *Beat Sugar Craving*, and *Healthy Parents, Healthy Baby*. She is the co-author of *No More IBS*, *Beat PMS Cookbook* and *Every Woman's Health Guide*. She has worked extensively on radio, including having her own weekly radio programme on health and nutrition, has co-written several medical papers and has written for many glossy magazines and for national daily newspapers. She has also appeared on many TV programmes on all five channels, radio programmes, had a regular page in *House & Garden* and *Healthy Eating*, is a regular contributor to *Good Health* magazine and is on the Board of Advisers for *Top Sante* magazine. She frequently lectures to both the public and the medical profession. She is married to Dr Alan Stewart; they live in Lewes, Sussex, with their four children.

Also by Maryon Stewart

Beat the Menopause Without HRT

No More PMS

Beat Sugar Craving

Healthy Parents, Healthy Baby

Co-author

No More IBS

Beat PMS Cookbook

Every Woman's Health Guide

Maryon Stewart's

Zest For Life Plan

Beat Fat and Boost Your Energy

Maryon Stewart

HEADLINE

First published in 1998
by HEADLINE BOOK PUBLISHING

10 9 8 7 6 5 4 3 2 1

ISBN 0 7472 5970 4

Typeset by
Letterpart Limited, Reigate, Surrey

Printed and bound in Great Britain by
Mackays of Chatham plc, Chatham, Kent

HEADLINE BOOK PUBLISHING
A division of Hodder Headline PLC
338 Euston Road
London NW1 3BH

To Gloria Newhouse,
my treasured old friend 'Down Under'

Contents

Acknowledgements

More than anything I would like to thank my wonderful patients over the last fourteen years, who have given me the clinical experience and the insight to write a book that has the potential to help millions of other people around the world get back into good physical and mental shape. Some of my more recent patients volunteered to share their stories, which involved divulging personal details, in the hope of helping others, and for this I am extremely grateful.

The hundreds of doctors and scientists around the world, who have been involved in research into holistic health and obesity, must be acknowledged, as many of their publications have been used over the years to develop the Women's Nutritional Advisory Service Programme, upon which this book is based. In particular I am grateful to Professor John Garrow, former Professor of Nutrition at St Bartholomew's Hospital, London, for his permission to use the chart on page 82.

I am grateful, as ever, to my dedicated team at the Women's Nutritional Advisory Service for their help and support. Special thanks are due to Helen Heap for her help with the menu and recipe section, to Cheryl Griffiths for her organisational abilities and typing skills, and to Allison Day for her important statistics.

Thanks are also due to Lavinia Trevor, my literary agent, for her sound advice that comes from years of experience, and to

Susan Fleming, my editor and friend at Headline, for her wisdom and perception.

I couldn't have written a single page without the support of my patient and caring nanny, Clare Fitzgerald, or that of my wonderful husband, Dr Alan Stewart, who cooked delicious meals and uttered words of encouragement and science to keep me on the straight and narrow.

Finally, I must thank my four children, Phoebe, Chesney, Hester and Simeon, for setting their needs aside and encouraging me to complete my task, so that I could spend some quality time with them during their school holidays.

Maryon Stewart

Introduction

In recent years dieting has become a dirty word in the nutritional profession and, in many ways, rightly so. There is truth in the rumour that 'dieting makes you fat' and the world would probably be a better place if books on weight loss – particularly the 'get thin fast' books – were banned.

Billions of women around the world are dieting at this moment in an attempt to improve other people's perception of them, and to revive their energy levels. And a recent Taylor Nelson poll/survey in America showed that one in three men is so unhappy about the size of his stomach that he would consider cosmetic surgery. It is fair to say that, as a race, we have been brainwashed to believe that skinny is desirable and healthy. But both of these premises are false, as you will come to realise.

Despite the fact that in January each year the media attempt to seduce us with even more 'new' methods of restricting our intake of food, an international effort to halt the worldwide obesity epidemic has recently been launched. According to the World Health Organisation (WHO), 'obesity is rising sharply and the current management or prevention strategies are not capable of arresting this epidemic'. Here are some pertinent facts:

- In the UK alone it is estimated that one in four people is overweight to some degree.

- In the USA and Canada one-third of the adult white

population is currently judged to be obese, and one estimate is that, on present trends, the entire population of America will be obese by the year 2234!

- Australia and New Zealand follow in the polls.

- According to a Risk Factor Prevalence Study Management Committee Report prepared in Canberra in 1989, obesity in Australia increased between 1983 and 1989 by 15 per cent for women and slightly more for men, bringing the totals to 11.1 per cent for women and 9.3 per cent for men.

- The Australian Institute of Health & Welfare's unpublished report of 1993 estimated the direct cost of obesity in 1988–9 at Aus$672 million, with obesity-related coronary heart disease and hypertension accounting for 62 per cent of that amount. The cost of treating obesity within the health-care system was Aus$393 million.

- European countries also score highly in obesity terms, and even in developing countries obesity is becoming a problem.

One could be forgiven for wondering how these trends have come about, when millions of people all over the world begin weight-loss diets each year. Booksellers fill their shelves with new diet books that they hope will catch the wave of New Year resolutions, and millions of hopeful, unsuspecting people fall for the hype.

The bare facts are that in the Western world we have been persuaded to go off the rails by greedy food producers and advertising agencies. Our increased prosperity has led us to over-indulge in the wrong sort of foods and drinks, which often contain chemicals and toxins that would make Mother Nature shudder, and to leave exercise to the likes of Cindy Crawford and Elle McPherson.

In truth, extensive research confirms that most people who follow weight-loss diets regain that weight, plus more, within a relatively short space of time, which makes the whole exercise entirely futile. The reason is scientifically based. Whilst dieting, our metabolic rate (the rate at which the resting body can burn up the fat we consume as food) falls with our diminished calorie intake. When we have reached our target weight and return to our usual way of eating, our metabolic rate remains at a reduced level, so our usual intake of calories becomes too great to maintain the weight loss. Hence the conclusion that dieting makes you fat.

Lack of knowledge about the actual requirements of our body leads us, as the years pass, not only to pile on the pounds, but also to acquire unwanted symptoms. There is no doubt that the diet most of us in the Western world eat as we enter the twenty-first century affects our mood, our energy levels and our zest for life, and will contribute to many of the unpleasant and serious illnesses to which we will succumb later in life.

During fourteen years of research and clinical experience at the Women's Nutritional Advisory Service (WNAS), where we actively help women with their health problems, we discovered that once we had established the right kind of diet and lifestyle for an individual patient, those who were overweight not only overcame their symptoms, but lost weight naturally as well, *without dieting*. In fact, many of our patients were eating far more than they had done before, and had thrown their calorie-counting books away. Without dieting, those who were 10 per cent overweight lost 3.6kg (8 lbs) within three months, and those 20 per cent overweight lost just under 5.8kg (13 lbs).

We have discovered, too, through research on women of childbearing age, that they very often have nutritional deficiencies that affect their brain's chemical metabolism. As the brain's chemistry can be likened to the conductor of an orchestra, in that it orchestrates different departments within the body, it follows that deficiencies have a knock-on effect on all body processes. Being short of vital nutrients often affects our immune system, the department of the body responsible for fighting off toxins. When this system is impaired or reacts to chemicals present in the food chain, it may mis-identify certain foods and drinks as being 'toxic', creating a chemical (antibody) reaction that causes havoc. The resulting symptoms may be either mental or physical, and include fatigue, loss of vitality, bowel disorders like constipation and diarrhoea, plus headaches, mood swings, food cravings, depression, loss of libido, panic attacks and palpitations. Chemicals can also cause the body to retain fluid, which then prevents the bathroom scales from registering any weight loss, even when on a low-calorie diet.

In the last decade it has become apparent that the number of individuals suffering from conditions like irritable bowel syndrome, chronic fatigue and food intolerance is on the increase. We estimate that at least 50 per cent of the women we treat at the WNAS experience bowel disturbances, such as constipation, diarrhoea, abdominal wind and bloating. Even larger numbers of people seem to be suffering from fatigue, and we commonly find that, whilst in a nutritionally depleted state, many suffer from what we call 'transient food intolerances' – transient because, once we have corrected nutrient levels over a period of months, and thus given the immune system a boost, we can then reintroduce the offending foods, often without any on-going reaction.

Although there is currently a lack of scientific information to explain precisely why common health problems are on the increase, after treating tens of thousands of women successfully over the years, it is our observation at the WNAS that a combination of nutritional deficiencies and the chemicals in our food – which our bodies were not designed to deal with – are probably responsible to a large degree. When individuals become familiar with their body's requirements and are more discerning about their choice of food, these actions invariably have a normalising effect on brain chemistry, which in turn helps the immune system to function normally. It is like flicking a light switch: the symptoms disappear, vitality and good humour return, and weight loss occurs in those who are overweight. Interestingly, those who are underweight seem to gain weight, which leads us to believe that when you discover the correct programme for your own body, it apparently has a normalising effect on your metabolism.

Through our work at the WNAS we have discovered that there is no substitute for education about the body's require-ments, in terms of both diet and lifestyle. It is a subject we miss out on throughout our education process, and this conspires to have dire consequences on our physical and mental well-being, and that of our families.

Whilst there is absolutely no place on the bookshelves for another diet book, there is undoubtedly a need to inform individuals about how to tune into their body's needs and be discerning about health choices. The results we have witnessed at the WNAS over many years are nothing short of spectacular.

Not only do we break through the weight-loss barrier, virtually without trying, but we also help to overcome unwanted symptoms and improve long-term health prospects. Within a matter of months we regularly transform individuals who are overweight, out of condition and feeling extremely unwell into people who are fit, trim, healthy and happy. Their self-esteem rises beyond their wildest dreams, and the effect this has on their relationships with sexual partners and children is positively satisfying for all concerned.

This book will provide the education that you have missed and will give you insight into cleaning up your act. Following its instructions will allow you to work out the best plan for your own health in both the short and long term, depending on your needs. It will give you the tools to interpret the messages that your body is sending, so that you can improve your general health and well-being at the same time as shaping up.

I have divided the book into four distinct parts. Parts One and Two look at how the 'diet trap' originated and at what's gone wrong with our diet and lifestyle as we approach the twenty-first century. They also show you how to assess your own situation and nutritional needs. Part Three provides the secrets of the WNAS plan, with suggested menus and recipes. Part Four gives brief advice for the long term, and is followed by appendices containing recommended reading, useful addresses and telephone support lines.

As women are usually considered to be the nutritional head of the household, it is vital that they soak up the missing facts about diet and lifestyle in order to help themselves and their families, and prevent their children from wandering even further off the path to good health. In this book I have attempted to translate fourteen years of experience into a workable plan to help you, your partner, your children and, I hope, *their* children. Make good use of the information – it's a gift from the WNAS.

The A–Z of Success Stories

This is the ninth self-help book I have written over the last ten years. In each book I have invited some of the WNAS's past patients to share their stories, in an attempt to reassure readers that there *is* light at the end of the tunnel. The response to these 'case histories' has shown their value: I continually receive letters from gratefully reassured individuals all over the world, and my clinic patients use the case histories as a source of inspiration whilst they are following the WNAS diet programme.

So here is an A–Z of success stories, which will demonstrate the power of the programme.

Arthritis

Jane Crighton, a Sussex postmistress, reports – 'Since I was fourteen I have experienced daily palpitations, which I thought I would live with for ever. When my menopause arrived I was overwhelmed with hot flushes, which I pretty much expected, and swollen painful joints, which I hadn't bargained for. Twenty-four hours after seeing Maryon Stewart for the first time, the palpitations had virtually ceased, which I thought was miraculous. Within weeks I was able to hold a pen comfortably; after a few months I had no more swollen painful joints and no more hot flushes. I feel so well – better than I can ever remember.'

Breast tenderness

A sore tale from Justine Hammond in Milton Keynes – 'I suffered from extreme breast tenderness premenstrually for seventeen years after the birth of my second child. They would start to swell and grow some seven to fourteen days before my period was due and gradually became so uncomfortable that I had to physically hold them when I moved. I read about the work of the WNAS and decided to contact them for help. Within a couple of months of starting my programme, my breasts felt easier. I simply don't have any breast tenderness at all now.'

Candida

From Annette Harris, a mum and student from Leeds – 'Thanks to all concerned at the WNAS. Without your tremendous support I would have continued to be overweight and feeling like death warmed up, tormented by chronic symptoms of candida, stress, anxiety and loss of libido. I'm now well, happy and one stone lighter.'

Depression

A thirty-year-old computer analyst in Essex, Joan Hart – 'I had been suffering from overwhelming depression and fatigue for over two years, and one memorable day I drank some alcohol at a work lunch and subsequently told my boss to get lost. Until then I had been a respected computer analyst and programer. I was at my wits' end, and didn't know where to turn for help. Miraculously, I was given a book written by Maryon Stewart, which made great sense, and my husband took me to see her. Within three months I was transformed into a happy, balanced, normal person. I'm still full of energy. We are out every night and I've become a sailing instructor.'

Eczema

A scratchy story from Scotland from Carla Castle, a mother of three – 'I read about the WNAS in a magazine, but it took me two years to summon up the courage to make contact with them. They put me on their programme and told me to eat lots of vegetables and fresh fruit, and to eat plenty of fresh fish. I had to cut out chocolate, caffeine and wheat. At first it was very difficult, but now it is just part of everyday life. I also took supplements. It only took me about four to five weeks before I was looking, and feeling, substantially better. I learnt that my eczema is particularly sensitive to diet, and that stress plays a part as well.'

Fatigue

From Glenda Smart, a schoolteacher from Wales who retired because of ill-health – 'I was unable to attend work because of my migraines and bilious attacks, and eventually took early retirement. I read an article in my local paper about the WNAS and contacted them for help. It was a wonderful experience – the whole programme made so much sense. The presentation and information were excellent and the programme helped me enormously. My symptoms, including constipation and fatigue, have disappeared completely and I'm back to my usual weight.'

The Gallops

Jane Masters, a teacher and Head of Year from Sussex – 'I think I could have got into the *Guinness Book of Records* for diarrhoea. I was really in trouble, passing explosive, frothy motions without any warning. My embarrassment was acute, as I worked as a schoolteacher, and I often had to run off and leave the children. Despite being given the medical "all clear", I was convinced I was terminally ill. My doctor just said it was due to irritable bowel syndrome (IBS) and that I'd have to learn to live with it. This was difficult, as it was ruining both my work and my social life, especially as I had PMS too, which drove me to swear like a trooper! My mum heard about the WNAS. I didn't need any persuading to make an appointment. Maryon Stewart gave me what seemed like a 5,000-mile service and a programme to follow. Within two months my symptoms were under control and after six months I had no diarrhoea whatsoever, no IBS, no PMS and no swearing! I'm now well, relaxed and happy and have had a lovely baby daughter since.'

Halitosis

A delighted shopkeeper, Julia Monk, from Wiltshire – 'I brushed my teeth several times a day, flossed between them, gargled with mouthwash, and chewed and sucked fresh-breath sweets and gums, and still I had foul-smelling breath, which left me feeling very humiliated and self-conscious. I was used to being such a lively and out-going person, but it's hard not to be inhibited when you are trying to keep your mouth firmly shut! I sent for the WNAS questionnaire and was stunned to see that bad breath was one of the subjects they asked about. I discovered that once I had tidied up my diet, and avoided certain foods, the bad breath cleared up completely. It's now ten years since I kissed bad breath goodbye, and it's wonderful to be able to smile and chat without having to be self-conscious.'

Irritable bowel syndrome

A mother and housewife, Jade Dench, who lives in Switzerland – 'Apart from complaining of IBS and regular sneezing fits, I had gained 15.75kg (35 lb) and, despite trying all sorts of diets, I couldn't keep the weight off. I read about the WNAS programme and flew to England to investigate. It's the best thing I ever did, and I now realise that I would never have got back to good health and been able to sustain the weight loss without finding the right programme for my body.'

Junkaholic

An ample mother of three, Jenny Millington, who is a library assistant – 'Chocolate was my biggest downfall. It was horrendous. I'd eat any kind of chocolate, including cooking chocolate, if there was no alternative. I used to feel extremely guilty afterwards, especially when I had eaten all the children's sweets, particularly their Easter eggs or selection boxes at Christmas. I was like a wild woman, capable of doing anything. I used to feel I would die if I didn't have my "fix". I felt irritable and edgy. Once I had eaten the chocolate, I would feel as if a great load had been lifted from my shoulders – and probably ended up round my hips! I used to get dizzy and light-headed. I followed the WNAS programme and noticed a difference within a month. Now I feel normal and not like a demented person.'

Knackered

A two-year saga of ill-health from Judith Lines – 'I tried everything – calorie counting, Weight Watchers, the Cambridge Diet, you name it. I used to sleep during the day because I was so tired, and I couldn't work because I didn't have enough energy. I was two stone overweight when I began the WNAS programme. I had headaches for the first three days, and I felt very irritable. I discovered that coffee gave me the shakes and made me feel very jumpy, and that foods containing yeast gave me a continual tummy ache and drained my energy. I actually felt that I had more to eat on this diet than on previous diets, yet I still managed to lose weight. I feel 100 per cent better now. I don't sleep in the afternoons any more, and the aches and pains have disappeared. I have much more energy – in fact I now go out to work.'

Loss of libido

Caroline Bennett, now Contented from Coventry – 'As much as I loved my husband, for seven years after the birth of our last baby I'd totally lost interest in sex. I simply felt that my husband's advances were an added aggravation, which of course placed great strain on our relationship. It was on one of my black PMS days that I saw Maryon Stewart on GMTV talking about improving your libido. My ears pricked up and I contacted the WNAS immediately. I started the programme that month and had my first symptom-free month two months later. My libido returned gradually and we have now reached the point where my husband is not sure if he can cope with this new woman.'

Migraine

Denise Pemberton, a sufferer from Wales – 'Following a very stressful period in my life when we lost three relatives in quick succession, my migraine headaches became constant. My GP tried me on HRT as I was approaching the menopause, but it made no impression on the symptoms, so after four months I stopped taking it. I contacted the WNAS for help after reading an article on their work in the *South Wales Echo*. I made gradual improvement during the first few weeks of following the WNAS programme and within months I felt so much better. I now only get the occasional mild headache, have so much more energy and am sleeping better. Additionally, two symptoms I had suffered from for years, swollen ankles and burning eyes, have cleared up completely. I certainly wish I had known about the WNAS a long time ago.'

Nausea

A London barrister, Ilanda Moore, describes a nightmare – 'It was like someone jerking a knife into my stomach. I'd be doubled over with pain and I'd always have to spend the first day of my period in bed. I'd experience nausea and be physically sick, and my abdomen would bloat out of all proportion. I found it very difficult to function properly at work. In fact I was only normal for seven days per month. I read about the WNAS and went along to their London clinic. I was asked to follow a very restricted diet initially, which was pretty tough, and to take supplements and to exercise. Within the first month, to my utter amazement, I had no pain. The nausea went as well as the bloating. I just couldn't believe it. That was ten years ago and I haven't had any period problems since. I am able to relax my diet, but I know that if I go back to my old ways, my symptoms will start to return. This programme was a complete cure for me; it totally revolutionised my life.'

Osteoporosis

A tale from Joanne Simms in Toronto – 'I had a surprisingly early menopause in my early forties, and was shocked to discover through a bone-density scan a 7 per cent bone loss in one year. It was therefore suggested that I take long-term medication for the osteoporosis. I'd never been keen on drugs, so I read Maryon Stewart's book *Beat the Menopause without HRT* and decided to give myself a year of natural solutions before accepting the drugs. Maryon helped me to refine my programme, which consisted of making significant dietary changes, taking nutritional supplements and daily weight-bearing exercises. The follow-up bone-density scan one year later showed virtually no further bone loss, so the consultant advised me to "keep taking the tablets". I'm hoping that next year's scan will show that I have made some new bone. I'm certainly feeling well, and much fitter, as a result of this new regime.'

PMS
A Sussex doctor, Nardine Baxter, conquered her symptoms of seven years – 'My father used to shout and have a bad temper, and I had a secret fear that I was beginning to develop like him as I grew older. Despite being a doctor myself, premenstrually I was inherently and constitutionally not a very nice person any more. The WNAS programme drove away "the witch". I'm back to my old self, feeling fit and slimmer too, plus I'm able to achieve more in life and enjoy my relationships. The success of the WNAS programme has been documented time and time again, and I now recommend it to my patients.'

Quest for sanity
An account from Josephine Hill, 'negative' in Sussex – 'I'd almost lost the plot and I came very near to losing my family. I suffered from terrible depression and mood swings, I was crying constantly and I felt negative about everything.

I was awake most nights, had zero libido and had all but alienated my husband with my constant nagging and complaints. We had been sleeping in separate rooms for some time anyway, then he left and I went into shock. I realised how low I'd sunk and how desperately I wanted the real me back. Fortunately, a friend recommended the WNAS. I went straight to see Maryon Stewart, who gave me a thorough overhaul. Her programme really reached the parts I'd neglected. Within days my lifelong constipation had gone and, as the weeks passed, I returned to inhabit my body. I became positive, rational, calm and relaxed. My husband could see a remarkable change in me each time he came to see us, and we were able to find solutions to our problems. In a short time he returned to us and a normal, much more settled family life. After all the doctors' opinions and their mostly unsuccessful theories, I still find it incredible that we did it all just through diet, exercise and non-drug supplements. Thank you.'

Recurrent infection

A report from Valerie Prince, a mother of two at a low ebb in Bristol – 'I'd got into a low state over the years and was really abusing my body as a result. I'd binge in secret and then experience palpitations and panic attacks. I'd actually been having panic attacks since I was fifteen. As a result of bingeing, I'd put on lots of weight. I used to pick up every infection going and go down with every bout of flu. Since following the programme Maryon Stewart wrote for me, I have made slow and steady progress. During the following winter I managed to stay well when everyone else went down with a vicious flu bug, which demonstrates that my immune system has had a great boost. I've lost weight and the panic attacks have diminished for the first time in my adult life.'

Stress

The potted history of Kathy Haynes, a mother of three and finance manager from Newcastle-upon-Tyne – 'I became so stressed out and forgetful as my menopause approached that I really believed I was in the early stages of Alzheimer's. I suffered from depression, mood swings, severe migraines, anxiety and confusion, which made it very difficult for me to continue to work full-time and concentrate on my degree course. In desperation I contacted Maryon Stewart for help and am delighted to say that, thanks to the WNAS and the support of my family whilst I followed the programme, I now live a full and happy life. I can hardly believe the person back there was really me.'

Thrush

Jacqueline Willis, a full-time mum and part-time sales assistant from Middlesex – 'I suffered from vaginal thrush for over a year and then developed a fungal infection on my neck and in my armpits. My doctor referred me to my local hospital, but the treatment didn't seem to make any significant difference. I was also undergoing hospital treatment for acne, which had developed after the birth of my second child. I felt very depressed and was finding it increasingly difficult to sleep at night. I contacted Maryon Stewart for help after seeing her on television. Within four months of following the WNAS programme I had no sign of thrush or any fungal infection. My skin is 100 per cent better, I've lost the excess weight I had and

I feel so much happier and much more relaxed. And, of course, my husband is delighted.'

Ulcers

A tale from Paula Wells, a Kent window dresser with two children – 'I used to suffer from mouth ulcers before my period, and then for three years the outbreaks became more frequent, to the point where I thought they might be related to something in my diet. I also suffered from PMS and IBS and was 3.2kg (½ stone) over my usual weight. A book I read on hormone health listed the address of the WNAS, so I decided to contact them for advice. That was in January 1996. I was given a programme to follow and within two months my bad days felt like good days used to feel, and the mouth ulcers had gone. By June I was feeling really well and had lost that unwelcome weight. During this process I discovered that lapses of eating wheat or chocolate brought back the old symptoms, including the ulcers. I now know how to keep well, and that feeling of well-being is motivation itself.'

Vitality

A weighty problem for Sue Cole, a London mother and housewife – 'I tried any diet that I could lay my hands on. I did lose weight but found that it returned as soon as I resumed my normal diet. Whilst dieting I used to skip breakfast and as a result felt unwell. I was always looking for a short-term miracle. I was awful to my husband and son. I realised I had to do something about it myself. I began the WNAS diet. It took me four to five months to get back to the weight I was before I was pregnant. I lost 12.7kg (2 stone) in all. I lost about 450–575g (1–1¼ lb) per week steadily after the initial weight loss. I felt so much better on the diet. I no longer had cravings for sweet or spicy food. I was calmer, nicer to my family and much more like my old self. I found that the caffeine in coffee was contributing to my feelings of nervous tension. As soon as I cut out brown bread, my stomach cramps went and all my unpleasant bowel-related symptoms went also, as well as my headaches, sore tongue and dandruff. I feel far more contented and in control now. The WNAS diet has taught me what foods suit me most. I have much more energy. I walk two miles a day and I have taken up gardening again.'

Weight loss

A report from a Yorkshire lass, Sandra Laws, who took part in a pilot project we conducted at the Nuffield Hospital in Huddersfield – 'For years I'd experienced unpredictable mood swings, to the point where my husband and kids hid from me whenever I was on the rampage. I'd been constipated for as long as I could remember and regularly had outbreaks of thrush and such painful periods that they put me in bed for days. Within two months of following the WNAS programme I had overcome all my health problems completely, and lost 5kg (11 lb) in weight. My husband can't believe the transformation after years of misery, and doesn't even seem to object to me buying loads of new clothes!'

Xcellent results!

The experience of Sally Crisp, a Sussex mum – 'I was pretty desperate to lose weight. I cut out fizzy drinks and chocolates for five months but I didn't manage to lose any weight. I felt hungry, miserable and frustrated. I used to get through seven or eight big bottles of cream soda per week and at least three chocolate bars per day, as well as sweets and sugar in tea. Looking back now, I realise my diet affected my moods. I used to hit out at my husband and throw things at him. I felt so upset with myself that I used to go out for a drive to cool off. I found the WNAS programme took some getting used to for the first few weeks. Once I got used to the diet, however, it was plain sailing. I lost 12.7kg (2 stone) in weight over a four-month period, and the weight loss has been maintained. What kept me going was reading about people who had been successful on the WNAS programme and seeing them on TV. I found I could not tolerate sweet foods, or foods containing whole wheat or yeast very well, and soon after I eliminated them from my diet I felt much better. Apart from the weight loss, I feel much more relaxed. I swim a lot and walk much more. In general I feel happier with myself at 54kg (8½ stone), and I feel I am able to get more out of life.'

Yo-yo dieter

Ups and downs for Mavis Wells, a housewife from Somerset – 'I had been on weight-reducing diets for many years without too much success. After starving myself to lose a few pounds, I would either get bored with the diets or get to feeling ill because of them. When I started the WNAS programme I had a few headaches at the beginning and later had a slight reaction to yeast and alcohol. I found that I managed to lose weight easily and I felt very satisfied on the diet. I now feel healthier, as well as feeling psychologically better for having lost the excess weight.'

Zombie status

A nurse from Sussex, Sue Cleasby, who previously described herself as a raving loony – 'I was like a zombie, who ranted and raved at everyone for three weeks of the month, to the point where I felt I was going mad. I tried all known cures and then one day I read about the work of the WNAS. I could hardly believe that a change of diet plus exercise could so radically change my life, but it has. I'm now sane every day and have regained my zest for life. I have a new career, and a very happy family. What more can I ask from life than being able to be me and not the monstrous woman I used to be.'

These are just a few examples showing the success we have had with the WNAS programme, on which this book is based. The benefits take a little while to become evident, so you will need to be patient; but, as you can see, it is worth persisting!

Part One

Diet and Lifestyle

Chapter 1

Who Set the Diet Trap?

The desire to be slim is nothing new, but in the past it never reached the fever pitch it has in recent years. Although there are no images of fat Stone Age people or Ancient Egyptians, as far back as 460 BC it was recognised by Hippocrates, the Greek 'father of medicine', that chronically ill patients who were unable to exercise, but maintained their dietary intake, lost their body shape. His recommendations even then for the overweight were to reduce calorie intake, to fast periodically and to pay visits to the gymnasium!

Early communities engaged in hard physical labour, and maintained both their shape and their fitness. Widespread weight problems did not seem to become an issue until the time of the Roman Empire, when the rich and powerful enjoyed orgies of over-indulgence. Many emperors and their families became so bloated that some of them had to be carried around by their slaves. Even then, prosperity was the root cause of obesity.

Changing values

In many of the centuries that followed, the problem was not obesity, but how to get enough to eat. By the fifteenth century, although no-one really knew what the optimum size (depending on height and build) for an individual was, advice about eating and drinking in moderation was beginning to be given by some physicians. But it was a layman, Luigi Cornaro, who really demonstrated the value of healthy eating and exercise. He rose from his deathbed, severely overweight at the age of forty, contrary to the advice of his physicians, and decided to throw away his medicines. Instead he ate approximately 350g (12 oz) of food per day and drank 400ml (14 fl oz) of liquid, and spent much time walking around Venice to improve his physical well-being and stimulate his mind. At the age of eighty-three, Cornaro wrote the equivalent of a bestselling book about his methods, and as a mark of his success he outlived his doctors and survived to see his *102nd birthday!*

The next major breakthrough came in about 1600, when one Dr Santorio Santorio, who was familiar with Cornaro's book, invented a hanging chair, the first weighing scale on record. He was fascinated by diet and body weight, and as a result weighed himself, his food, drink and excrement for thirty years. He also recorded his physical and sexual activity, in an attempt to determine how much food the body actually used.

From one extreme to the other

In the decades that followed, it is fair to say that the rich were generally fatter than the poor. Women at that time were far from preoccupied with their weight, as it was generally considered desirable to be plump. Seventeenth-century artists like Peter Paul Rubens used models who weighed 88–100kg (14–16 stone), such was the appeal of the ample, voluptuous figure. So how did we get from 'fat is beautiful' to where we stand today, at the other end of the spectrum?

It was in Victorian times that the concept of women's shapeliness began, and men set about providing whalebone corsets to pull in the waistline. Even then, though, being thin was still undesirable to suitors, as it was associated with infertility. But by the end of the First World War it was becoming fashionable and elegant for women to be slim. The trend continued, much to the delight of many profiteers. In 1925 certain disreputable doctors like Dr Yves Latimer and Dr Gabriel Leven claimed to be able to reduce weight by giving sub-cutaneous injections and hot baths, and even suggested giving up fluids completely for an unspecified amount of time. The most extreme treatment tried in the late 1920s was electric shocks, which were thought to stimulate muscle activity.

By the 1930s the diet industry had been truly launched, with countless pills and potions that would 'guarantee' weight loss. Manufacturers claimed there was no longer a need to diet by conventional means, and of course there was no shortage of customers. This dangerous trend was alleviated to some degree by the foundation of the Women's League of Health and Beauty, which spread the concept of healthy eating and exercise across most of Europe. Sadly, the good work it did became diluted over the years, by the images portrayed in advertising agencies and the media. 'Twiggy' set one tone for the new look in the 1960s, which has continued to this day with the current vogue for 'waif' models. Have you ever seen an 88kg (14 stone) model in a magazine or television commercial?

Thankfully, pills and potions are somewhat out of fashion these days. What has replaced them are books on how to lose weight quickly, many of which appear authoritative. Rapid weight loss, however, is not a good long-term solution. It is far better to get to know your own body's needs and to find the diet and lifestyle programme that is uniquely right for you. But first, we need to examine the numerous factors that influence our food choices and learn how to read the messages that our bodies send us.

Chapter 2

Where Diet Took a Wrong Turn

The power that diet, environment and lifestyle have on our health is awesome. Before even considering how it may influence us as adults, it is important to realise that the health of a sperm and an egg, four months before conception, will determine the health of the unborn child, not only in infancy, but also throughout adult life – including whether that individual will be predisposed to heart disease, stroke, asthma or other chest complaints. Isn't that staggering?

There is, however, a great deal we can do to help ourselves to better physical and mental shape during our lifetime, and it is almost never too late to start. Being aware of the changes that have occurred to diet and lifestyle in recent decades will at least give you some insight into the situation.

Food for thought

In the last fifty years as society has changed (and not necessarily for the better) diet and lifestyle have altered dramatically. At one time culinary skills were passed on from one generation to the next, and the woman very definitely played the 'home-maker' role. She was not expected to go out to work whilst her family was growing, and more often than not she had her mother and other female relatives living close by as back-up. The motor car was a luxury, so her daily shopping was usually done locally on foot. She would expect to purchase fresh food regularly, which would contain far more nutrients than produce purchased weekly from the supermarket. As fast food didn't exist, part of her role would be to cook wholesome meals for the family on a daily basis.

Fifty years on, the picture is quite different. Women have learned the art of the short-cut, very often through necessity. They drive to the supermarket once or twice a week to purchase food and are presented with pre-prepared, fast-food choices which, when short of time and adequate information, seem both convenient and appealing. Most of the food they buy has been preserved, sprayed with chemicals, injected or indeed grown in chemically rich soil. That food has been treated with pesticides and insecticides, and animals pumped full of antibiotics and growth hormones, is almost taken for granted, and environmental pollution is merely the cherry on top.

But human bodies were not designed to be treated in such a fashion, nor to cope with modern-day stresses, so it is no wonder that we develop health problems. We probably treat our domestic appliances or our car with more respect than we do our bodies. Few of us would dream of denying our car the appropriate fuel or oil, so how is it that we neglect our bodies so? At the WNAS it is our experience that a lack of education is responsible, for when individuals are confronted with the real facts about diet and lifestyle, they usually take action. Once enlightened, few of them revert to their old habits, as they are so pleased with the renewed health they experience and surprised at how enjoyable their new diet and lifestyle are. As an added bonus, they are able to pass their new-found knowledge on to other members of their family.

Impoverishing our diet

Let us examine more closely how our eating habits have changed. A century ago, meat, animal fat and sugar formed a much smaller proportion of our diets than it does today. On the other hand, the consumption of cereal fibres has actually dropped considerably.

- We have increased our consumption of sugar. The UK has become one of the world's largest chocolate- and sweet-eating nations, currently spending over £5 billion per year on chocolate alone. Australians and New Zealanders consume on average 50kg (110 lb) of cane sugar per person per year.

- Sugar consumed in packaged and processed foods has increased from 30 to 70 per cent over the past fifty years. And the last 100 years have seen a 25-fold increase in world sugar production. In reality, refined sugar is not something that we actually need, and the human race managed quite happily without it for centuries. Mother Nature, with her usual wisdom, designed it so that the body can convert complex carbohydrates and proteins into the sugar it requires. Table sugar, or sucrose, actually contains *no* vitamins, minerals, protein, fibre or starches; it may contain tiny traces of calcium and magnesium, if we are really lucky, but otherwise all it provides is 'empty calories'.

- We have to go out of our way these days to reduce our sugar consumption, as 'considerate' food manufacturers often add it to the most unlikely foods: cheese, fruit yoghurt, tomato sauce, baked beans, pickled cucumbers, muesli, beefburgers, Worcestershire sauce, sausages, peas, cornflakes and canned drinks, to name but a few.

- Excessive consumption of saturated animal fats results in a gradual blocking of the arteries that supply the heart, brain and other major organs. This leads to poor circulation, then to heart attacks and strokes. It is worth noting that smoking accelerates this process. The increased incidence of breast cancer has much to do with animal-fat consumption as well.

- We eat far too much salt – ten to twenty times more than our bodies really require each day – which can contribute to high blood pressure.

- We often drink far too much coffee and tea, which can impede the absorption of essential nutrients and aggravate symptoms of nervous tension, irritability, insomnia and headaches. On average we consume four mugs of tea and two mugs of coffee each day, which deliver approximately 800mg of caffeine into our system. That doesn't include other sources of caffeine, like chocolate, cocoa, cola and other caffeinated drinks. It certainly means that there are many people walking about with symptoms of caffeine excess. Count how many mugs you have had today – you may be surprised.

- We consume volumes of foods containing a high level of phosphorus, which impedes the absorption of beneficial nutrients, and interferes with calcium absorption by bone tissue. Examples of these foods are soft drinks (low-calorie or normal varieties), processed foods, canned, packaged, pre-packed convenience foods and ready-made sauces.

- Alcohol consumption has almost doubled in the UK since the end of the Second World War. This too impedes the absorption of beneficial nutrients, and in excess alcohol can cause all sorts of other health problems (see chapter 10).

- Unbelievable as it may seem, we actually eat less food now than we did thirty years ago. It seems that today's generation actually expends less energy than our grandparents' generation, which has resulted in a 10–15 per cent reduction in food intake. This has also meant that our intake of essential nutrients has fallen, particularly if refined or convenience foods are being eaten.

- Many foods available today contain chemical additives in the form of flavour enhancers, colourings and preservatives. While a number of these are not harmful, some of them are, and our bodies are certainly not designed to cope with them.

- These days our meat animals are bombarded with antibiotics, to the point where the animals often become resistant to them. The antibiotics are used as a preventative measure, and often for growth promotion, but can have adverse effects on our bodies when we consume the meat.

- Nitrate fertilisers have been used to obtain fast-growing and abundant crops. It is now recognised that nitrates are harmful and can produce cancer, at least in animals.

- Almost all our fresh fruit, cereals and vegetables are sprayed at least once with pesticides. In addition, milk and meat may retain pesticides from feed given to livestock, as you will discover in more detail in chapter 6.

Whilst it is deeply depressing that the quality of much of our food is out of our hands, increased insight will undoubtedly help us to make better choices. Including wholesome and freshly cooked food into our diet rather than processed or pre-prepared varieties will make for a good start. It's worth questioning older generations of the family about their shopping, cooking and eating habits in earlier years. Combining the best of old habits with the outstanding variety of foods we have to choose from today is likely to be a winning combination.

Chapter 3

A Diet to Make You Sick

You may wonder just how much effect our modern diet has on metabolism and nutritional status. My doctor husband and I wanted to put this to the test, so we set up an experiment to measure the effects that alcohol, cigarettes, sugar, tea and coffee have on the balance of nutrients in the body.

The experiment

Alan, my husband, who is usually in excellent nutritional and pretty good physical shape, was the guinea pig. (Fortunately, we did not have to fight over it, as I was breastfeeding at the time.) His usual diet is above average nutritionally, he was not taking any supplements and is a non-smoker. He is only a moderate consumer of alcohol, sugar, tea, coffee and chocolate. The aim of the experiment was to see what effect consuming the national average amount of these 'toxins', plus cigarettes, would have on this fine healthy specimen.

Two weeks before the experiment began Alan's blood levels of vitamins and minerals were measured, and were all well above the normal range. They were measured again at the start of the experiment and every two weeks during the 'active' phase, which was due to last for eight weeks.

As well as his usual diet, Alan had to consume the following each day:

tea – 4 cups

coffee – 2 cups

alcohol – 3 units (1 unit = 1 glass of wine, 1 measure of spirit or 300ml/½ pint of beer or lager)

chocolate – 1 small bar (approximately half a large Mars bar)

soft drinks – ½ can of cola

sugar – 12 teaspoons (i.e. 2 teaspoons in each of the hot drinks)

cigarettes – 6

The tea was made according to the instructions given by the Tea Council in London, brewing the teabag for three minutes, then squeezing it. The cigarettes were smoked properly, with each being inhaled as much as possible!

The first week

I felt quite apprehensive about this experiment and wondered what it would be like to live with Alan whilst he was being our guinea pig. I also felt some concern about whether, in eight weeks, Alan might develop a taste for the alcohol, the chocolate or even the cigarettes!

The first few days were very trying for Alan, as he went on the new regime suddenly rather than gradually. He had previously drunk hardly any tea, only one or two cups of coffee without sugar per day, had the occasional alcoholic drink and smoked only the odd cigar. He developed quite a severe migraine headache, felt very sick by Day 3 and was on the verge of giving up. However, as he had made a start, he was determined to continue, come what may . . .

The second week

During this time Alan felt very run-down. He developed a flu-like cold, which lasted for several days. This was most unusual, as he is rarely ill. And he found that he was so full up from all the liquid in his diet that he hardly had room for his evening meal. His usual hearty appetite for three courses was reduced to the point where he was pushing his main course around his plate complaining that he felt nauseated and tired.

The calories provided by the extra alcohol, sugar, and chocolate were some 500 to 600 per day, and as Alan did not gain weight during the experiment, we knew that his intake of beneficial foods must have fallen by approximately 20 per cent, compared with his normal daily intake.

The third week

Alan is usually a very even-tempered individual who has endless energy. He is often perky until at least midnight. By the third week, however, he was nodding off to sleep in an armchair as soon as he had finished dinner and by 8.30 pm could not be roused. He also developed a slightly more aggressive attitude, and became a bit short-tempered at times. He was still experiencing the nausea, especially after smoking. Constipation was also becoming a problem – he just couldn't eat the amount of fruit and vegetables he had tucked into before. And the tea and coffee with two teaspoons of sugar in each were not helping. By the time he had drunk them, mainly in the morning, his stomach was rumbling and churning like a cement mixer.

The fourth week

By this time Alan's libido had begun to wane. His usual enthusiasm had definitely disappeared; more often than not he was asleep anyway. Our former lifestyle was fast becoming a memory, and I was really wondering whether the experiment had been a good idea after all.

The fifth week

I now seriously wondered how Alan was going to manage to keep going for another four weeks. I was particularly worried about him after an evening out in a restaurant: he had been getting behind with his alcohol intake, so he decided to catch up. He consumed a bottle of Frascati and smoked two cigarettes, then turned green, almost passed out and fell asleep sitting up in the chair.

Although the laboratory was not meant to divulge any results to Alan until the eight-week period was over, I decided that it might be better to know the results at six weeks and perhaps bring the experimental diet to an end at this point. Alan agreed that six weeks was probably enough, partly because he did not think he could manage to continue for another two.

The sixth week

By this time Alan was feeling pretty ill. He was very tired and found it hard to concentrate for long periods of time. One lunchtime, after consuming his ration of junk food and two cigarettes, he fell asleep on a sofa in his waiting room with a can of cola in his hands. When his first patient for the afternoon session had to wake him up, he knew it was definitely time to abandon the diet. Fortunately the patient saw the funny side of the situation!

The laboratory results

It was just as well that Alan did decide to finish the diet after six weeks, as it turned out that many of his vitamin and mineral levels were sinking very fast. The laboratory results on individual nutrients were as follows.

Vitamin A

Alan's vitamin A levels fell by nearly 50 per cent in six weeks. Vegetable vitamin A 'carotene' fell by 30 per cent, and both levels were now at the lower end of the normal range. Vitamin A is necessary for healthy vision and resistance to infection, and a good intake reduces the risk of cancer. Deficiency usually occurs only in the presence of a grossly inadequate diet or when severe digestive problems exist.

B Vitamin group

Vitamins B_1 (thiamin), B_2 (riboflavin) and B_6 (pyridoxine) were measured. From their normal, healthy levels at the start, mild deficiencies of all three developed after just six weeks. B-group vitamins are necessary for protein and energy metabolism. Deficiency can affect mood, energy levels, skin quality and resistance to infection.

Vitamin C

Alan's vitamin C levels fell rather dramatically, from the top end to almost the bottom end of the normal range by the end of the six-week experimental diet. This level was by no means low enough to cause scurvy, as Alan was still eating fruit and vegetables, albeit less than before. Interestingly, the first symptom of vitamin C deficiency is depression. Smokers are known to have lower vitamin C levels than non-smokers, and it was probably smoking that most affected Alan's vitamin C level.

Vitamin E

His vitamin E level also fell by some 30 per cent, from the middle to towards the bottom of the normal range. This level would have had to fall much further to produce a deficiency, however, and would be unlikely to occur in anyone unless they were eating a very poor diet indeed.

Zinc

This important mineral also fell slightly by some 15 per cent. No deficiency developed, which is just as well, because zinc has important functions influencing sex hormone and sperm production, resistance to infection and appetite.

Magnesium

Magnesium levels fell by 10 per cent. Again, no deficiency developed, and the fall was almost certainly caused by the reduced intake of green vegetables, a major source of magnesium, and by the increased losses from the body that can occur through alcohol and coffee consumption. Magnesium is needed for the energy-producing steps in normal metabolism.

Chromium

The blood level of this mineral also fell, from a very good, healthy level to the lower end of the normal range. Chromium helps to control blood sugar and cholesterol levels in the body. A high sugar intake, which was part of Alan's diet, greatly increases the loss of chromium in the urine. It is thought that high sugar intakes and low chromium levels predispose to hardening of the arteries and raised cholesterol levels in later life.

Selenium

This mineral dropped by 15 per cent during the six weeks. This small fall did not produce a deficiency, which is anyway rare in a normal, well-fed, population. However, those who have lower levels of selenium may have an increased risk of cancer in later years. The same seems to be true of vitamins A and E. The best food sources of selenium are fish and whole grains.

What did all this mean?

We were both pretty devastated that in just six weeks, eating and drinking these commonly consumed substances could have had such an appalling effect on Alan's nutrient levels – whilst he was eating a healthy diet as well! We knew that he was feeling awful and behaving in an uncharacteristic manner, but we did not expect the fall in nutrient levels to be so great in such a short space of time.

Certainly the average consumption of alcohol, cigarettes, sugar (and possibly even tea, coffee and chocolate) does not help our nutritional balance. People vary enormously in how their bodies tolerate these dietary items, and in Stage 2 of the diet you will learn how your body gets on with some of these items.

What happened afterwards?

At the end of the sixth week Alan stopped taking the cigarettes, sugar, tea and the extra coffee, alcohol and chocolate. Within three days he felt that he had been born again. Only then did he fully realise that he had been experiencing a mild dull pressure in the head, as well as nausea, and physical and mental fatigue.

For the next eight weeks Alan went back to his old diet – again, not taking any supplements. During that time, all his vitamin and mineral levels were restored and Alan once again enjoyed good health, apart from another cold two weeks after stopping smoking and drinking.

Conclusion

What does this rather unusual experiment show? First, it is difficult, if not dangerous, to argue that what happens in one case happens in all. It does not. Some people can smoke heavily and drink significant amounts of alcohol, and get away with it.

We know that it is easier for your body to tolerate the habit if you also eat well, but many people do not. Others feel ill just at the smell of cigarette smoke or even a small glass of wine.

We are all different, but it is certainly possible that for many of us our current consumption of cigarettes, alcohol, tea, coffee, sugar and even chocolate is enough to affect our health and our nutritional balance adversely. Even an average consumption of these can be harmful to us. For many people, reducing consumption – or even stopping all of them for a while – is likely to help in a number of ways. For example, some 25 per cent of calorie intake is on average derived from alcohol and sugar. As these are very poor-quality foods, they really form no significant part of a healthy eating plan. Consumed in small quantities as part of a healthy diet (once your weight is normal), they probably do no harm, and their pleasures are of course well known. More details about alcohol, sugar, tea, coffee, chocolate and cigarettes are given in chapter 10.

So we have seen how ill an average consumption of these common 'foods' can make one person feel. In Part Three we will see how much better you could feel by avoiding them. Remember: the aim is that you should not only lose weight, but, more importantly, feel really healthy, with your body in good nutritional balance.

Chapter 4

Getting the Balance Right

Our bodies were not designed to survive healthily for very long on a diet composed of any one type of food. Not only would this be monotonous, it would also fail to provide the range of nutrients required for health, including proteins, fats, carbohydrates, vitamins, minerals and fluid. Whilst I am sure you have come across all these terms before, no nutritional book would be complete without laying out the bones of a balanced diet.

What's essential?

Proteins

These are the building-blocks of the body. They are essential for health and, unlike fats and carbohydrates, cannot be reduced significantly without resulting in adverse effects both in the short and in the long term. Proteins are composed of long chains of building-blocks known as amino acids. There are twenty or more of these, some of which are essential, some non-essential. The essential amino acids include isoleucine, leucine, lysine, methionine, phenylalanine, threonine, tryptophan and valine, and these need to be obtained from dietary sources as they cannot be manufactured by the body. The non-essential amino acids include aspartic acid, glutamic acid and tyrosine, and these can be synthesised in the body.

Proteins are divided into two groups. First-class proteins, which contain significant quantities of all the essential amino acids, can be found in meats, fish, eggs or dairy products. Second-class proteins, which contain some of the essential amino acids, are vegetable proteins from foods like beans, nuts, lentils and seeds. It is therefore more difficult for a vegetarian diet to provide the complete range of amino acids.

Tissues, such as muscle, heart, liver, kidneys and most other organs, are rich in protein. Skin, bones and hair also contain certain amounts of protein, which contributes to their structure. The main role of proteins, however, is to support the functions of each individual cell. Thus protein is necessary for the ovaries and thyroid to produce hormones, for the kidneys to make urine, for the muscles to exercise, and so on. If a large amount of protein is consumed in the diet, then some is used for energy purposes and, during starvation periods, protein is taken from the muscles of the body and used as a fuel supply. This tends to slow down the body's metabolic rate, and for this reason weight-loss diets should include plenty of protein. On average for every 6.4kg (1 stone or 14 lb) of body weight, we require a daily intake of 5g (⅛ oz) of protein (about half an egg). This is essential to keep the body healthy.

Carbohydrates

Carbohydrates come in a variety of different forms, all of which are best regarded as sources of energy. The simplest forms of carbohydrate in our diet are glucose and fructose. These are single-sugar units, and fructose is found in particularly high amounts in fruit, hence its name (which means fruit sugar). Fructose and glucose can be joined together to make sucrose, or table sugar, normally prepared from sugar cane or sugar beet. Milk contains yet another type of sugar called lactose, which is itself composed of two single units of sugar, glucose and galactose.

So much for simple carbohydrates. Complex carbohydrates, which are found in vegetables, cereals and to a lesser degree in fruits, are composed of numerous sugar units joined together in a more complex way. These have to be broken down by the digestive system before they are absorbed as single units of mainly glucose and fructose. Complex carbohydrates are desirable for three reasons:

- they are slowly digested and release their energy at a steadier rate than simple carbohydrates

- foods rich in complex carbohydrates are also rich in vitamins and minerals, which are essential for the metabolism of sugar and the steady release of its energy

- such foods are also full of fibre, high intakes of which are associated with many health benefits.

Refined carbohydrates, such as sucrose and pure glucose, may be a convenient source of quick energy, but they lack vitamins, minerals and fibre. They are all too easily consumed to excess, and thus may lead to obesity.

Fibre

This is a specialised form of complex carbohydrate, which cannot be broken down by the normal human digestive system. It thus becomes a major constituent of the waste product, faeces. A diet rich in fibre helps to prevent conditions like constipation, diverticulosis and other digestive troubles, as well as coronary artery disease, gallstones and appendicitis. Fibre-rich foods are generally filling and satisfying as they often require a considerable amount of chewing, and they are also usually nutritious. A diet rich in fibre from green leafy vegetables will provide you with large quantities of vitamins A, B, C and E, as well as magnesium and a wide range of other minerals. A tablespoon of bran, which may provide you with the same amount of fibre, is not nearly so nutritious.

Overweight people tend to consume less fibre than their normal-weight counterparts. Those who are overweight tend to have higher levels of fats in their blood. Fibre-rich foods, combined with weight loss, can help to reduce fat levels, thus lowering the risk of heart disease.

Fats

Fats are a major source of energy in the diet, and provide twice as many calories as protein or carbohydrates for the same amount of weight. In developed countries, fat intake has increased at the expense of a reduction in complex carbohydrates, and in order to lose weight, we almost always have to cut down on our fat intake. Some fats, however, are essential, just as vitamins and minerals are. These are the polyunsaturated fats, which are derived mainly from sunflower, safflower and rapeseed oils, vegetables, nuts, seeds and some fish.

Foods of animal origin – for example, lard, dripping, butter, milk, cream, cheese and meat, and some vegetable oils (notably palm oil and coconut oil) – are rich in saturated fats. These are not essential in the diet, and have the undesirable effect of stimulating the liver to produce more cholesterol, thus raising its level in the blood. (Both saturated and polyunsaturated fats contain the same amount of calories.)

ESSENTIAL FATTY ACIDS – These essential nutrients – known as EFAs – are needed for the health of the nervous system, skin and blood vessels, and they also help to keep our hearts healthy and to control inflammation. They consist of two key groups, the Omega-3 EFAs (which can be found in cod liver oil, mackerel, herring and salmon oils, and soya bean oil), and the Omega-6 EFAs which are present in sunflower, safflower and corn oils, evening primrose oil and many nuts (excluding peanuts), seeds and green vegetables.

CHOLESTEROL – This is a specialised form of fat, which is found particularly in eggs, dairy products and meat. Most of the cholesterol in our blood is actually made by the liver, and approximately one-third is derived from our diet. Dietary cholesterol is not the ogre the experts once thought it was, and in fact we now know that there is 'bad' LDL-cholesterol and 'good' HDL-cholesterol. The body needs some fats, but saturated animal fats, especially when combined with a lack of fibre in the diet, should be avoided.

Approximately 15 per cent of our diet is composed of protein, 45 per cent of carbohydrate and 40 per cent of fat.

Vitamins and minerals

These are essential nutrients, required not for their calorific value, which is negligible, but because they assist in normal functioning of the thousands of different chemical reactions that make up the body's metabolism. If their supply in the diet is inadequate, this will result in changes in body chemistry and a slowing down or altering of the body's metabolism, usually alongside some deterioration in body fitness or health. Vitamins and minerals often work together in this respect and are necessary for normal energy production, the use of protein in growth and tissue repair, as well as many other functions, ranging from hormone production to skin quality. Additionally, some minerals – particularly calcium, phosphorus and magnesium – are necessary with certain types of protein for the maintenance of the body's skeletal structure.

ANTIOXIDANTS – The main antioxidant nutrients are vitamins A, C and E and the minerals selenium, zinc, manganese and copper. Their function is to kill off the free radicals which are scavengers within the body that, given the chance, damage our cells and fur up our arteries. A regular intake of antioxidants is important as they protect us against cancer, heart disease and premature ageing.

Several foods contain plenty of the antioxidant nutrients, including green and yellow vegetables (spinach, broccoli, Brussels sprouts, carrots and red peppers), and garlic and onions.

A well-balanced diet

An important part of a healthy weight-loss programme is getting the nutritional balance right. On average, we have an excessive intake of calories derived from fat and carbohydrate; protein intakes are normally adequate, unless the diet is very restricted; and, if we are eating a healthy, well-balanced diet, our intake of vitamins and minerals is almost certainly adequate, but how many of us are truly eating such a diet?

At certain times of our lives, and in certain situations, it may be difficult to achieve a proper balance of all the vitamins and minerals in the diet. These situations include:

- episodes of rapid growth, such as puberty

- pregnancy

- breastfeeding

- prolonged or heavy periods

- prolonged adherence to a weight-loss programme

- adherence to a very restricted, or fad, diet

- adherence to a vegetarian or vegan diet, unless it is well balanced

- old age

- periods of taking long-term drugs, such as steroids, diuretics, anti-epileptic drugs and possibly the oral contraceptive pill.

If you fall into any of the above categories, you may need to take a daily multi-vitamin and mineral pill as your nutritional insurance policy (see chapter 11).

Vegetarian diets

These are becoming increasingly popular, and indeed can be very healthy. By definition, vegetarians do not eat meat or fish, but may include eggs and dairy products (milk, cheese, butter, and so on). Strict vegetarians who avoid even these foods are called vegans.

The main difficulty with vegetarian diets is ensuring a good intake of protein, and of the nutrients such as iron and zinc that are found in protein-rich foods. Meat and fish, as well as eggs and dairy products, provide a balance of amino acids, the essential components of proteins. Plant foods, however, do not, unless two or three different plant foods in the diet are combined, preferably at each meal. Particularly good combinations are:

- rice, with legumes (pulses), sesame seeds or cheese

- rye with legumes

- Quorn with mixed nuts and milk

- wheat with sesame seeds and soya bean

- corn with legumes

- mixed nuts with sunflower seeds.

The most protein-rich members of the legume family are, in declining order: mung beans, red kidney beans, haricot beans, butter beans, chickpeas, red pigeon beans, lentils, peas (fresh or frozen) and split peas.

Adding 300–600ml (½–1 pint) of milk and one egg each day to a vegetarian diet generally increases its protein content and makes it easier to achieve a nutritional balance using plant proteins.

Chapter 5

Interpreting the Body's Messages

Bodies are highly complex 'machines' that are designed to be efficient and are brilliant at communicating. The problem is that we are not taught 'body-speak', so we usually ignore the messages they send us, as we have little idea of how to interpret them. In fact our bodies have very specific requirements in order to function efficiently, and women in particular have varying needs throughout the many phases of their lives. Nutritional requirements at puberty are quite different from those during pregnancy, for example, and differ again from the demands made at the time of the menopause.

Changing body needs

The following lists will give you some idea of the changing nutritional needs of the body during the different phases of life and at times when common conditions present themselves.

Note that where animal protein is mentioned, vegetarians should include a wide variety of vegetable protein, such as legumes, Quorn, soya, nuts and seeds (see page 240 for the start of the vegetarian recipes).

Stages

PUBERTY – All nutrients, and particularly iron, zinc, calcium and magnesium; plenty of fresh fruit and vegetable fibre; regular wholesome meals; reduced amounts of animal fats and refined snacks like chocolate and cola-based drinks.

PRECONCEPTION – Folic acid; other B vitamins and EFAs; healthy, wholesome diet in the form of regular meals and unrefined snacks, such as unsalted nuts, dried fruit, cereal bars, etc.

PREGNANCY – All nutrients, particularly EFAs; a wholesome diet in the form of regular meals; regular snacks of fresh fruit, unsalted dips, home-made cakes and biscuits using fruit, ground almonds and cooked egg.

BREASTFEEDING – EFAs; calcium, magnesium and iron; a wholesome diet similar to that outlined for pregnancy.

MENOPAUSE – Calcium, magnesium, vitamin E; EFAs; foods containing the naturally occurring hormones such as oestrogen, known as phytoestrols (plant oestrogen), like soya, linseed, almonds, green and yellow vegetables, sprouted beans; plenty of oily fish, salad and fruit; reduced amounts of caffeine, alcohol and spicy foods, as these aggravate hot flushes.

POST-MENOPAUSE – Calcium, magnesium; EFAs; vitamin D, if deficient; phytoestrols (see menopause); plenty of oily fish, fruit, salad and vegetables.

THE ELDERLY – Vitamins B, C and D; calcium and iron; regular wholesome meals containing fresh fruit, vegetables, salad, oily fish and both soya and dairy products.

Conditions

ACNE – A strong multi-vitamin and mineral supplement, with extra zinc; eat regular wholesome food, concentrating on fresh fruit, vegetables and salad; a minimum of animal fats and sugar, including chocolate, alcohol and fizzy drinks containing chemicals.

CONSTIPATION – Supplements of magnesium up to your gut tolerance; organic linseeds with non-wheat-based cereal daily; plenty of fresh fruit and vegetable fibre; lots of fluid; low tea consumption.

DIARRHOEA – A strong yeast-free B-complex; no wheat, bran or dairy produce, coffee, alcohol or spicy foods.

FATIGUE – A strong multi-vitamin and mineral supplement containing vitamins A, C, E and zinc; marine fish oil and evening primrose oil; a wholesome, magnesium-rich diet that contains plenty of fruit, vegetables and salad (particularly green leafy varieties); regular intake of protein; reduced consumption of wheat and bran, plus restricted amounts of caffeine, alcohol and refined snacks like chocolate.

HEAVY AND/OR PAINFUL PERIODS – Multi-vitamins and minerals with extra B vitamins; vitamin C with bioflavonoids and magnesium; EFAs; plenty of green leafy vegetables, oily fish, liver, free-range eggs and other foods rich in iron and magnesium.

MIGRAINE – Yeast-free multi-vitamins and minerals; supplements of magnesium and feverfew; none of the amine foods, like cheese, chocolate, alcohol, pickled foods, tea, coffee, citrus fruit and monosodium glutamate; regular meals; and chew some ginger, either crystallised or root.

Nutrient	Food sources	What they do
Vitamin A	*Retinol (animal vitamin A)* Liver, all dairy products and margarine *Beta-carotene (vegetable vitamin A)* All yellow, green and orange fruits and vegetables	Essential for vision, especially in the dark, for growth and resistance to infection
Vitamin B$_1$	Meat, fish, nuts, whole grains and fortified breakfast cereals	Essential for the metabolism of sugar, especially in nerves and muscles
Vitamin B$_2$ (riboflavin)	Milk, meats, fish and vegetables	Involved in energy release from fats and carbohydrates
Vitamin B$_3$ (nicotinamide)	All forms of meat and fish, liver, fortified breakfast cereals and bread	For energy release from fats and carbohydrates, health of the skin and nervous system
Vitamin B$_6$	Meat, fish, nuts, bananas, avocados, whole grains	Essential for the metabolism of protein and the amino acids that control mood and behaviour. Affects hormone metabolism
Vitamin B$_{12}$	All forms of meat, liver, eggs and milk, yeast extract	Involved in the chemical functioning of the nervous system, and the blood cells
Vitamin C (ascorbic acid)	All fresh fruits and vegetables	Involved in healing, repair of tissues and production of some hormones
Vitamin D	Milk, margarine, sardines, cod liver oil, eggs (and sunlight)	For the balance of calcium in bones and teeth, and for muscle strength
Vitamin E	Most nuts, seeds and vegetable oils and dark-green leafy vegetables	Protects tissues from wear and tear, keeps cholesterol and other fats from deteriorating inside the body
Vitamin K	Green leafy vegetables, and the bacteria in our intestines	Helps with blood clotting
Folic acid	All green leafy vegetables, liver and fortified cereals	Helps maintain the health of the nervous system and the blood

Who is at risk	Symptoms	Visible signs
The ill, elderly and poorly fed pre-school children	Poor night vision, recurrent chest infections	None
Alcohol consumers, women on the pill, breastfeeding mothers, high consumers of sugar	Depression, anxiety, poor appetite, nausea, personality change	None usually! Heart, nerve and muscle problems if severe
Those on a poor diet. Deficiency rarely severe	Mild fatigue and possibly burning feet	Peeling of the skin on the lips. Red ring around the iris of the eye
Alcoholics, those on a poor diet, and with poor digestion	Diarrhoea, depression and dermatitis	A sore tongue and red scaly rash in light-exposed areas
Women, especially smokers, 'junk-eaters'	Depression, anxiety, insomnia, loss of responsibility	Dry/greasy facial skin, cracking at corners of mouth
Long-term vegans, those who have lost part of their stomach, and the elderly with digestive problems	Anaemia, loss of balance and a sore tongue	Smooth sore tongue, pale appearance, and unsteadiness
Smokers particularly	Lethargy, depression, hypochondriasis (imagined illnesses)	Easy bruising, look for small pinpoint bruises under the tongue
Urban-dwelling, dark-skinned immigrants, especially young children and pregnant women, those with little sunlight exposure	Softening of the bones, poor teeth and weakness of the hip muscles	Enlarged skull, bowing of the legs and a waddling gait
Those on a very poor diet, or with serious absorption problems	None. Damage to the nervous system if severe	None
Those with a poor diet or on long-term antibiotics	Prolonged bleeding	None
Those on a poor diet, those taking anti-epileptic medication, coeliacs, and a percentage of the normal population of childbearing women who are at increased risk of having a child with a neural tube defect	Often none. Possibly depression, fatigue and poor memory	None unless anaemic

Nutrient	Food sources	What they do
Iron	Meat, whole grains, nuts, eggs and fortified breakfast cereals	Essential to make blood-haemoglobin. Many other tissues need iron for energy reactions
Zinc	Meat, whole grains, nuts, peas, beans, lentils	Essential for normal growth, mental function, hormone production and resistance to infection
Magnesium	Green vegetables, whole grains, Brazil nuts and almonds, many other non-junk foods	Essential for sugar and energy metabolism, needed for healthy nerves and muscles
Calcium	Milk, cheese, bread (especially white), sardines, other fish with bones, green vegetables and beans	Needed for strong teeth and bones, also for normal nerve and muscle function. Lack leads to osteoporosis (bone thinning)
Potassium	All vegetables and fruit	Needed for the health of all cells, especially muscles and the nervous system
Selenium	Most wholesome foods, especially seafoods	Involved in two enzymes that protect inflamed and damaged tissues and help thyroid function
Chromium	All wholesome foods, not sugar and other refined carbohydrates	Helps in the action of insulin. Deficiency causes a diabetic-like state
Essential fatty acids Omega-3, fish and related oils	Cod liver oil, mackerel, herring, salmon, rapeseed and soya bean oil	Help control inflammation, reduce calcium losses in urine
Essential fatty acids Omega-6, evening primrose and related oils	Sunflower, safflower and corn oils, many nuts (not peanuts) and seeds, green vegetables	Control inflammation, needed for health of nervous system, skin and blood vessels

Who is at risk	Symptoms	Visible signs
Women who have heavy periods (e.g. coil users), vegetarians, especially if tea or coffee drinkers, women with recurrent thrush	Fatigue, poor energy, depression, poor digestion, sore tongue	Pale complexion, brittle nails, cracking at corners of mouth
Vegetarians, especially tea and coffee drinkers, alcohol consumers, long-term users of diuretics (water pills)	Poor mental function, skin problems in general, repeated infections	Eczema, acne, greasy or dry facial skin
Women with PMS (some 50 per cent may be lacking), long-term diuretic users, alcohol consumers	Nausea, apathy, loss of appetite, depression, mood changes, muscle cramps	Usually none, so easily missed; muscle spasms sometimes
Low dairy consumers, heavy drinkers, smokers, women with early menopause. Lack of exercise increases the rate of bone-loss calcium in later years	Usually none until osteoporotic fracture of hip or spine. Back pain	Loss of height
The elderly, after prolonged vomiting, with use of some diuretics and poor diet	Weakness, low blood pressure and muscle cramps	None
The ill elderly, those on a very poor diet, possibly those with heart failure or long-standing malabsorption, alcoholics	None that are specific, just general unwellness	None
The elderly, life-long consumers of junk food!	Those with diabetes or low blood sugar, or with episodic weakness and sugar craving	Perhaps a large waistline or sweet wrappers in their pockets!
Those on a poor diet, older people, diabetics, drinkers	None	None
Those on a poor diet, diabetics and drinkers. Also those with severe eczema and premenstrual breast tenderness	None	Possibly dry skin

Premenstrual syndrome – Particularly magnesium, B vitamins, iron and EFAs; plenty of fresh fruit and fibre; a daily salad; three portions of oily fish per week; low intake of caffeine, animal fat and refined snacks like chocolate, cakes and biscuits.

Thrush – A yeast-free multi-vitamin and mineral supplement; supplements of zinc and iron daily; supplements of the herbal product Uvacin; a low-yeast diet that avoids sugar and foods that contain sugar and alcohol, ensuring a regular intake of wholesome food.

Nutrient needs

In order to fully understand your nutrient requirements, you need to become familiar with the role of each individual nutrient, and with the signs of deficiency. The following tables will provide you with all you need to know – and a little more besides.

By now you should have a better idea of what your body is trying to communicate, and perhaps what it *doesn't* need on a regular basis, as well as what it has been crying out for!

Chapter 6

The Unsuspecting Consumer

Before our food reaches our plates, much of it is exposed to numerous chemical processes, and these days it may even be genetically engineered, or irradiated. This was not the case in the past, which may, to some degree, explain the increase of modern health problems like irritable bowel syndrome, eczema, chronic fatigue and headaches. Perhaps our food did not look quite so perfect years ago, but at least it was not tampered with by greedy conglomerates whose sole intention is to swell their profits.

The chemicalisation and pollution of our food is very much a political issue, and is kept under wraps by the food and farming industries. For years organisations like Friends of the Earth, The Food Commission and The Soil Association have been campaigning to ban the use of certain agro-chemicals in food, as they have been shown to be detrimental to human health. Although some agro-chemicals have indeed been banned, the warning messages have to a large degree fallen on deaf ears.

The use of agro-chemicals in the soil and of growth promoters in animal feed will ultimately result in a larger harvest and larger animals – which translates into increased revenue for farmers and the food industry at large. This would be all very well, were it not for the fact that these agro-chemicals cause harm to the environment and to our health. Our liver, kidneys and immune system were clearly not designed to be bombarded at regular intervals each day by residues of agro-chemicals and additional hormones.

When looked at in detail, this subject is pretty horrifying, especially as the consumer is effectively caught in a trap, unless he or she happens to be a fully self-sufficient smallholder!

Agro-chemicals – the facts and figures

Let's first examine some of the agro-chemicals that are used; then look at what we can do to avoid at least a few of them.

Pesticides

These come in three guises: insecticides which are used to kill insects; herbicides, which are used to kill or suppress the growth of certain plants; and fungicides, which are used to kill or suppress the growth of fungi. According to a 1998 Ford Commission report in Costa Rica, around 100 people die and 10,000 are severely poisoned each year by $55 million worth of pesticides drenched over Costa Rican vegetables and fruit destined for export. And, in Kenya, workers on pineapple estates spray pesticides banned in developed countries.

INSECTICIDES like organophosphates (OPs), which have recently been linked with Gulf War Syndrome, are compounds that are in fact diluted and modified nerve gases, which attack the central nervous system of insects and animals. They may be applied in the form of sprays or powders directly on to animals or pests, and are used in the soil to deal with problems like carrot fly. They are chemicals that are absorbed by plants and then eaten by insects.

Organochlorides (OCs), another type of insecticide, include

the well-known chemical DDT. These were initially thought to be safe, and were widely favoured as they were inexpensive. They are however persistent pesticides, which means that they are not broken down, but instead remain in the environment long after they have served their purpose. They are particularly attracted to fatty substances, and residues are often found in animal products like milk, cream, cheese, meat and human fat. Women usually have more body fat than men, and are therefore likely to store greater quantities of chemical residues.

Carbamates are naturally occurring substances, but are much more toxic than other organochlorides. Because of their low persistence, they present less of a problem to the consumer, and on occasions even have medical uses. They are often used as a last-resort pesticide, as they are twice as expensive as other insecticides.

HERBICIDES are used to kill off the weeds that would otherwise compete with crops for food and light. Some varieties just kill the weeds, others kill off plants, too. The most infamous of herbicides was 245T, which has now been banned in the UK as it causes vomiting, diarrhoea, burning pains in the mouth, and muscle weakness.

Other herbicides have caused inflammation to skin, dermatitis and blistering in severe cases. Our bodies were not designed to ingest these.

FUNGICIDES are used either to prevent fungal growth, or for the treatment of fungus on perishable foodstuffs. They are more commonly applied as a preventative measure, as they are long-lasting. This invariably means that some of our food is likely to contain residues, and indeed in the mid-1980s Thiabendazole was detected in the skins of lemons in the UK.

It is primarily used to protect stored potatoes.

Many of the pesticides still in use leave residues in our food, and these have been shown to be detrimental to human health. Our individual tolerance varies enormously, but it is fair to say that most of us would be hard pushed to escape being exposed to them to some extent. It is difficult to obtain exact statistics, but many of these substances precipitate allergies; some can affect the unborn child whilst it is developing, while others affect babies when they are being breastfed; and indeed some are classified as carcinogenic, which means that they cause cancer.

We also have to contend with the nitrates that are present in our soil, which are used as preservatives and fertilisers, resulting in residues in our water supply. And whilst we are assured by the suppliers that our water is safe to drink, containing no more than 40–50mg of nitrates per litre, a report prepared by the Food Commission in London in 1985 showed that seventy water supplies in the UK exceeded this level – and over one million people were using this water daily.

In themselves nitrates are not that harmful, unless you consume an enormous quantity; their main health hazard, however, is that they change into nitrites by a process of reduction, and nitrites are thought to be associated with increased rates of cancer.

Antibiotics, colouring agents and hormones

Not only have the animals we eat been fed foods that have been grown in chemically treated soil, and perhaps crops that have been sprayed, but they have often been treated with antibiotics in an attempt to reduce the spread of infection. Eggs are sometimes injected with artificial colourants to make the yolks look brighter; fruits are often sprayed and injected in an attempt to make them look more appetising and have a longer shelf life. Hormones continue to be used by farmers to increase milk supply and regulate egg laying. The residues from all of these drugs and chemicals find their way into our bodies, although the vast majority of people are unaware of their existence.

This massive subject is worthy of a book in its own right. The important thing is to be aware that much of the food presented to us is not as Mother Nature intended. The numerous processes involved in the rearing and growing of food mean a reduction in basic nutrition, and the answer must lie in organic food choices wherever possible. Although organic food is harder to obtain (unless you grow your own), and more expensive weight for weight, by consuming it you will be decreasing the number of agro-chemicals you consume, and thus increasing your nutrient intake. According to The Soil Association, organic vegetable foods are more nutrient-dense for the equivalent weight. As they have not been contaminated by chemicals, they deliver much more of what nature promised.

The same is true of meat. Additive-free or organic meat has not been subjected to drugs, growth promoters or contaminated foods. This type of meat is now far more widely available than before (even our local high-street butcher supplies it), and some local farms, and many supermarkets, keep stocks. If you find 'clean' meat, it can be included in your diet approximately three times per week, unless of course you are vegetarian.

Label liability

If you haven't already started reading food labels in the supermarket, have a go next time you go shopping; sadly, there are more than a few surprises in store. Make sure you have plenty of time to spare as many of the contents lists are pretty long, and although they give some information about ingredients, they don't give the detail really needed about quantities or chemical content. Alas, the new European law only requires information about key nutrients such as fats, salt and sugar if the product makes a health claim. A Government survey carried out in 1991 on 1,000 people showed that 50 per cent of consumers read labels and want more information, such as whether pesticides have been used, whether the animals were treated with veterinary medicines, whether the product has been genetically modified or irradiated, and the quantities of the main ingredients.

The Guild of Health Writers is currently running a campaign called FLAG (Food Labelling Agenda, see page 358 for details), in which it is calling on food manufacturers and retailers to provide clear and meaningful labelling so that we know what our food really contains and the processes to which it has been subjected. Campaigns will continue until we have achieved our right to know precisely what it is we are eating. Until that day, you will be armed with at least some useful knowledge about food safety by reading food labels, and we recommend that you make a point of doing so thoroughly. But remember, you can't beat a good meal that is home-made from fresh natural ingredients.

Fear or fare?

With the advent of 'mad cow disease' (BSE) in cattle, salmonella in eggs, *E.coli* and listeria in soft cheese and pâté, the last few years have seen many food scandals, which have caused a great deal of confusion and fear about which foods are really safe for us to eat. It is debatable whether the quality of our food has actually taken a nose-dive in recent times, or whether it is longer-term problems that have been exposed.

Whilst major food-safety campaigns over the last few years have not resulted in entirely safe food, they have reached the parts of public awareness that were not reached before. The proof of this is reflected by the statistics.

In the main, we are now more safety-conscious when it comes to what we eat, but confusion still reigns about what exactly is safe to keep on the menu. In 1990, a Mintel survey reported that the UK food industry had lost £250 million in the last few years because of food scares and scandals. The Food Safety Act 1991 offers a framework for legislation throughout the food chain – in other words, from the farmer to the supermarket. In theory, everything that can be eaten is protected by the Act, and indeed, some improvements have already come into effect. For example, the 'sell by' date on labels has been replaced by 'use by' dates for perishable goods such as soft cheese, fresh cream products and live yoghurt. And supermarket chill cabinets are now operating at lower temperatures than before, which protects high-risk foods like meat, cured fish, salad ingredients and sandwiches. Despite all this, in 1996 the Consumers Association tested fresh and frozen chicken and found that half contained either salmonella or campylobacter bacteria.

Realistically, BSE and salmonella contamination will not disappear for some time to come. Irradiation is on the increase and retailers are being very secretive about genetically engineered food. Monsanto, the American food giant, is churning out genetically engineered soya by the ton, and is quite determined that it will end up on our dinner tables. Despite numerous requests about which foods are likely to contain genetically engineered soya or corn products, the supermarkets are not particularly forthcoming. Equally horrifying is that current legislation does not require genetically engineered ingredients in foods to be identified as such on the food label. Outrage on the part of both the shoppers and the retailers has resulted in proposed new labelling laws which will mean that some genetically modified food will be identified, but by no means all. Soya oil for example, which is often listed as vegetable oil, and lecithin, the additive which is made from soya, will both be exempt. Consumer campaigns over the next few years will hopefully change this, empowering us once more with the freedom of choice that we have recently lost. For useful addresses, see page 357.

Whilst the campaigns for safer food continue, there is no substitute for becoming 'street-wise' about the food that we are consuming and serving to our loved ones. There are many protective steps that can be taken on an interim basis that will help you retain your health and sanity.

Practical measures

If you can't live without your Sunday roast, but are worried about the risk of BSE, then try to buy organically reared or additive-free beef. A good butcher or local farm should be able to give you information about the herds from which they draw their beef, and in many cases you will find that supermarkets now stock organic beef. Alternatively, many UK supermarkets now stock Australian steak and even kangaroo steaks, which make a delicious alternative.

- Always wash your hands with soap and water before handling any food.

- Trim the visible fat off meat before you cook it, as toxins accumulate in fat.

- Due to the over-fortification of animal feeds, liver and liver products like pâté and sausage may contain high levels of vitamin A, which can be toxic to an unborn child. If you are pregnant or contemplating becoming pregnant in the next six months, it is recommended by the UK Department of Health that you avoid these products altogether.

- Pâtés and soft, unpasteurised cheeses may contain the bacteria listeria, which can cause severe flu-like symptoms and may prove fatal to an unborn child.

- Cook-chill foods should be heated thoroughly before eating to kill off any harmful bacteria.

- Toxoplasma, a bacteria that can cause blindness in new-born children if acquired during pregnancy, can be found in raw meat, which should be avoided, especially during pregnancy.

- If you have a cat, keep it away from food and food preparation areas, especially if she has recently had kittens. Pour boiling water on to cat litter or any soiled area in the house. Cats are major carriers of toxoplasma.

- Wash fruit and vegetables thoroughly. They may be contaminated with surface bacteria.

- Make sure that you clean out the fridge regularly and that it is cool enough during hot weather.

Many individuals and organisations campaigned for additive-free food, and this is now fairly widely available, or at least we have a choice. Perhaps it is time to start campaigning again, this time for residue-reduced food – with enough consumer pressure, this could come about. In the meantime, getting yourself into good nutritional shape and consuming a diet that helps to boost your immune system will assist your body to deal with the agro-chemicals and other toxins that we undoubtedly ingest on a regular basis.

This book is designed to help boost the immune system, with a view to making you more resistant to the constant bombardment of agro-chemicals. Details of supplements that will help to boost the immune system are given on page 111.

How our food choices are influenced

Large food corporations and retail chains spend good money on psychologists' fees in an attempt to influence our food choices. It may sound bizarre, but their successful techniques have turned into a financial harvest at the expense of the unsuspecting consumer. Fast music, bright colours and a wide variety of choice – not to mention the sylph-like females who appear on the chocolate ads! – all encourage us to eat more. Being familiar with the tactics employed by these corporate giants at least gives us a fighting chance of taking control of the situation, rather than being herded along as just another gullible consumer!

Research at Johns Hopkins University in Baltimore revealed that those who listened to fast music whilst eating ate five large forkfuls per minute, compared to the three smaller mouthfuls eaten by those listening to slower music. The fast eaters were more likely to request seconds, as they reached the end of their serving before their body had a chance to register 'full'.

Another revelation from Johns Hopkins University, this time from the Weight and Stress Department, is that bright colours increase our appetite. This means bright-coloured foods (no wonder the food industry is loath to part with artificial colouring), food wrappings (no need to guess why chocolate bars are so boldly packaged), and brightly coloured décor, both on the outside and the inside of many fast-food chains.

Well-presented buffets also encourage us to eat more. And a study from Pennsylvania State University showed that human guinea pigs given four different courses ate 60 per cent more food than their counterparts who were given four servings of the same food. Translated into everyday terms, this presumably means that those who have a wide variety of foods on offer in their supermarkets will be tempted to eat more than their counterparts who have little choice!

Eating with family and friends, it seems, also encourages greater indulgence, regardless of the time of day and whether we are eating at home or in a restaurant. A psychology professor and his team at Georgia State University in Atlanta have repeatedly discovered from hundreds of seven-day-diet diaries that eating in company, rather than alone, results in 44 per cent more food being consumed. I wouldn't suggest for a moment that you give up eating in company as food and good company are two of life's great pleasures, simply be aware of the pitfalls!

Part Two

How to Help Yourself

Chapter 7

Assessing Your Needs

Getting to know your own body is a bit like learning how to use a highly complicated machine without a manual. It can be a difficult process and one that requires time and practice.

Each individual human body has a different type of metabolism (the chemical reactions that occur in each cell and organ to keep the body functioning normally) and slightly different requirements. The type of metabolism that we have is inherited. There are those lucky individuals who have a superbly adapted metabolism: they naturally have a low blood cholesterol level, can eat almost any type of food, in large quantities, and yet remain healthy and slim. It is highly unlikely that you are reading this book if you happen to be one of the fortunate few!

We have to come to terms with the fact that there are subtle differences that determine the strengths and weaknesses of our make-up. This explains in principle why some people are predisposed to illness or tend to be sensitive to certain types of dietary change, groups of food or nutritional deficiencies. This can also explain why, on an identical diet, some people get sick and overweight, while others remain slim and healthy.

General health

The purpose of this book is to give you the information you need to compile the nutritional manual that will tell you what is just right for your body. In order to be able to interpret your body's messages you have to learn to tune into the signs and clues that will eventually lead you to an understanding of your individual needs. With that in mind, I have gathered together a number of the WNAS's questionnaires for you to complete. This will help you to locate any trouble areas that require attention.

General health questionnaire

Let's start with a general questionnaire about your health. This will help establish whether any recent health problems you have had may be affected by your diet, or by alcohol and cigarette consumption. Score 1 point for a YES, no points for a NO.

Do you have, or in the last year have you had, any of the following?	YES	NO
Anxiety or depression requiring treatment by your doctor	❑	❑
Prolonged fatigue for no known reason	❑	❑
High blood pressure	❑	❑
Recurrent vaginal thrush	❑	❑
Repeated colds, coughs, sore throats or chest infections	❑	❑
Premenstrual tension	❑	❑
Difficulty conceiving	❑	❑
Repeated mouth ulcers	❑	❑
Gum disease requiring treatment	❑	❑

Do You

Smoke cigarettes regularly? ❏ ❏

Consume more than 14 units of alcohol per week (1 unit – 1 glass ❏ ❏
wine, 300ml (½ pint) lager, or 1 measure spirits)?

If you ticked two or more of these points, then it is time to take stock of the situation. Each of these common problems could be related to your diet, or to alcohol or cigarette consumption. Alternative reasons exist for these problems, of course, but improving the quality of your diet, and reducing your intake of alcohol and cigarettes if you consume them, must help with the problems – and for some people it could make a very big difference indeed.

If you have any of the conditions listed above, your doctor may already have spoken to you about the importance of healthy eating and a healthy lifestyle. If you are receiving medical treatment for any of these conditions (or for any other condition, for that matter) do check with your doctor before starting the WNAS programme or any other diet. There should not be a problem, but it is always best to check.

Heart disease

Now let us see what the future might hold. Heart disease and strokes remain two of the biggest causes of death in most developed countries and, more importantly, are perhaps the most preventable causes of premature death, before the age of sixty-five.

The following questionnaire is designed to give you some

idea of what your risk of heart problems might be. It is only a guide and should not be considered infallible. Certain factors, such as smoking, high blood pressure, diabetes, obesity and high blood cholesterol, increase the risk. Exercise and eating plenty of fish, fruit and vegetables are associated with a lower risk. Family factors can also be important, and anyone reading this book who has a first-degree relative (mother, father, sister or brother) who experienced a heart attack before the age of fifty-five should see their own doctor for a detailed assessment, no matter what they score on the questionnaire.

Answer each question carefully, then add up your score.

Heart disease questionnaire

	YES	NO
Do you smoke cigarettes?	3	0
If you are a non-smoker, have you smoked in the past 10 years?	1	0
Have you ever been diagnosed by a doctor as having a heart disease or a heart attack?	3	0
Has your mother, father, brother or sister had a heart attack or heart disease?	2	0
Are you a diabetic requiring insulin, specialist diet or drugs?	1	0
If you are diabetic, have you had diabetes for more than fifteen years?	1	0
Do you have high blood pressure, requiring treatment?	1	0

Is your blood pressure well controlled by treatment?	0	1

If you have had your cholesterol level checked, was it:

less than 5.2 millimols/litre?	0
between 5.3 and 6.5 millimols/litre	1
over 6.5 millimols/litre	2
not tested	0

What is your grade of obesity on the height/weight chart (see page 82)

grade 2 or 3	1
grade -1, 0 or 1	0

Do you exercise vigorously once or more per week, or walk for more than thirty minutes per day, every day?	0	1

For women:

Do you drink more than 3 units of alcohol per day?	1	0

For men:

Do you drink more than 5 units of alcohol per day?	1	0

For men and women:

Do you eat fish two or more times per week?	0	1

Do you eat fresh vegetables or fruit daily?	0	1

TOTAL SCORE

If your score is 0, 1 or 2, then this is pretty low, and if there is no family history of heart trouble at an early age it would appear that you are less likely than average to experience heart disease. A score of 3, 4 or 5 would suggest an average to slightly increased risk, when compared with the rest of the population. If it is smoking, being overweight or lack of exercise that produced this score, then it is obvious what you should do. Otherwise see your doctor (if you are not already receiving medical treatment), who can advise you about further risk factors, and check your blood pressure and cholesterol if necessary.

If you scored 6 or more – unless this score was produced by smoking, being overweight or lack of exercise – then you must definitely see your doctor. Indeed, it would be a good idea to see him or her before making a start on the programme in this book. If you are already under medical supervision because of high blood pressure or diabetes, then do discuss any points raised by this questionnaire that have not been covered by your treatment so far.

Chapter 8

Assessing Your Excess Baggage

Being overweight may be a mark of prosperity in a community used to food shortages, but for those of us who have food aplenty, our spare pounds cannot be viewed as a trophy of any kind. So let's not waste time dreaming up justifications; instead, let's get down to some hard facts.

Obesity defined

The graph below gives measurements for height and weight. It is divided into five sections, – 1, 0, 1, 2 and 3. These represent grades of obesity based on individual's weight and height, taken from a formula originally devised by the Belgian scientist, Lambert Adolph (Jacques) Quetelet.

Quetelet's Index, more usually known as Body Mass Index (BMI), is still widely used in the assessment of obesity today. The formula is derived by multiplying your height in metres by itself and then dividing your weight in kilograms by this figure, or:

$BMI = \dfrac{weight}{height^2}$ (See page 85 for metric conversions.)

Let's use my measurements as an example. I'm 1.65 metres tall, so that multiplied by itself equals 2.72. I divide my weight, which is 55.5kg, by 2.72 and the result is 20.4.

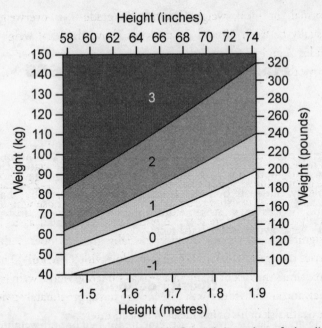

Height/weight chart showing the Quetelet grades of obesity

Unless you are brilliant at arithmetic, you will need to use a calculator. When you have your result, check it against the categories below.

Less than 20	Grade –1
20–25	Grade 0
25–30	Grade 1
30–40	Grade 2
40+	Grade 3

Normal, or ideal, weight is grade 0; grade 1 is overweight (usually between 10 and 20 per cent above the ideal weight); grades 2 and 3 are regarded as obese (more than 20 per cent above the ideal weight); grade –1 is underweight.

The health risks of obesity

As measured by the Body Mass Index, the range associated with the greatest life expectancy and lowest death rate is 20–25 (grade 0). There is a very slight rise in the death rate of those who are mildly overweight (grade 1), but this rise is so small as to be insignificant. It is grade 2, and especially grade 3, obesity that carries the greatest risk to health. An adult with a BMI of 40 has three times the risk of dying in a year as someone whose weight is ideal, and an individual with a BMI of 35 has approximately twice the death risk of his or her ideal-weight counterpart.

For most people who are just slightly overweight (grade 1 obesity), the major reasons for following the instructions in this book are to feel well and to look good. In this grade, there is little change medically in factors such as blood pressure and risk of heart disease due to weight, though there could be a moderate fall in blood-cholesterol level if this is elevated at the start of the diet.

For those with grade 2 or 3 obesity, the potential benefits of losing weight are very real, and the effects on the psychological state of an individual following a successful weight-loss programme can be dramatic. Those in this category have a shorter life expectancy, and an increased risk of many illnesses, including diabetes, high blood pressure, heart disease, osteoarthritis, gout, gallstones, a reduction in exercise tolerance and level of fitness, and depression. Furthermore, general medical problems may be more difficult to treat in those who are obese. Gastro-intestinal disorders, including indigestion, heartburn and constipation, may be harder to assess in an obese individual, as the information obtained from a medical examination may be limited. And the survival rate of the obese woman with breast cancer is lower than that of her slim counterpart.

The young obese individual who loses weight to reach normal or near-normal weight levels may enjoy a substantial improve-ment in their quality of life and life expectancy, and a reduction in risk in practically all of the above conditions. The improvement in arthritis, gout, blood pressure, diabetes or blood-cholesterol level may be dramatic and will be evident within a few weeks or months of starting the new dietary programme.

The underlying causes of obesity

Obesity tends to run in families. Research shows that if both parents are obese, 70 per cent of the children will be so, too. If one parent is obese, 40 per cent of the children will be; if both parents are lean, then only 10 per cent of the children will be obese. The predisposition of the parents is thus partially carried down to the children, but of course we could argue that obese parents eat too much and are thus likely to over-feed their children, making them obese in turn, and that this has nothing to do with genetics or inheritance.

However, studies of children who have been adopted show that they follow the weight characteristics of their biological parents, rather than those of their adopted parents. This and other work lends substantial support to the theory that the tendency to obesity is, to a large degree, genetic.

Environmental factors play a significant part as well. By 'environment' we mean all the factors that occur around us and potentially influence our internal metabolism, which is initially determined by genetic make-up. The most important environmental factors associated with obesity are food supply, level of exercise, lifestyle and social pressures.

If food supply, for example, is so meagre that there is barely enough to go round, or starvation conditions exist, then obesity will obviously disappear from the community at large. In such a situation, environment plays a greater role than any genetic factor. However, when there is an abundance of food, exercise and lifestyle are the environmental factors that may keep obesity in check.

The only practical solution to an ever-growing obese population is to change the eating habits of those who are overweight, while taking other steps to improve their rate of weight loss.

Recognising obesity

No-one wants to admit to being obese, but if you feel that you have a weight problem, look at the very approximate height/weight guidelines given below, and recognise that *now* is the time to do something about it, before your health begins to suffer.

WOMEN	HEIGHT	MEN
Weight without clothes	(without shoes)	Weight without clothes
	6 ft 4 in/1.95m	181 lb/82.1kg
	6 ft 3 in/1.92m	176 lb/80kg
	6 ft 2 in/1.89m	171 lb/77.6kg
	6 ft 1 in/1.87m	116 lb/75.3kg
152 lb/69kg	6 ft/1.84m	162 lb/73.5kg

WOMEN	HEIGHT	MEN
148 lb/67kg	5 ft 11 in/1.81m	158 lb/71.7kg
144 lb/65.4kg	5 ft 10 in/1.78m	153 lb/69.4kg
140 lb/63.5kg	5 ft 9 in/1.76m	149 lb/67.6kg
136 lb/61.7kg	5 ft 8 in/1.73m	145 lb/65.8kg
132 lb/60kg	5 ft 7 in/1.70m	140 lb/63.5kg
128 lb/58.1kg	5 ft 6 in/1.68m	136 lb/61.7kg
123 lb/55.8kg	5 ft 5 in/1.65m	133 lb/60.3kg
120 lb/54.4kg	5 ft 4 in/1.62m	130 lb/59kg
116 lb/52.6kg	5 ft 3 in/1.60m	127 lb/57.6kg
113 lb/51.3kg	5 ft 2 in/1.57m	123 lb/55.8kg
110 lb/50kg	5 ft 1 in/1.55m	
107 lb/48.5kg	5 ft/1.52m	

If you are 20 per cent or more above these figures, it is important to ask your doctor to check your thyroid to see whether it is underactive. And it is advisable to ensure that you are not suffering from diabetes or high blood pressure. If any of these checks are positive, they will need addressing by conventional medical means.

Chapter 9

Curbing the Cravings

One difference between fat people and thin people is that thin people's bodies tell them when they have had enough to eat. Fat people's bodies just don't know when to say no. Certain factors switch the appetite on or off. If it is too readily switched off, we become underweight; if it is too readily switched on, we become overweight. It is not yet fully understood how the appetite is controlled: hunger, caused by lack of food, is the most obvious and indeed most powerful stimulus, but often we have an appetite even though we are not very hungry. In such circumstances, the sight, smell or, indeed, taste of food and drink serve to stimulate our appetite. Something looks delicious, we have eaten it before and know that it tastes delicious – and hey presto, we have an appetite for it. Many of us also eat to comfort ourselves when we feel stressed or emotionally upset.

Social circumstances dictate eating habits and appetite as well. It is customary to offer a drink or snack to guests and, in some circumstances, it is impolite for them to refuse. Indeed, you have probably broken previous weight-loss diets because of social pressures, such as eating out in a restaurant, or dining at a friend's house where their encouragement ('Go on, it won't hurt') and your response ('Just this once') are the first fatal steps to weight gain.

Certain drugs, including some sex hormones, antidepressants and steroids, serve to stimulate appetite. Emotional factors, in particular recovery from depression, and sometimes response to depressive episodes, may also result in an increased appetite.

So much for what switches appetite on; what, if anything, switches it off? The sensation obtained from a meal, including abdominal fullness and an inner feeling of satisfaction, sometimes mingled with the horror of further weight gain, does usually switch the appetite off. Physical or emotional pain, illness and some drugs also tell us that now is not the time to eat.

A further important factor is body image. Some people of normal weight feel that they are grossly overweight and must diet to obtain a 'normal' body shape. Their image is to some degree distorted, and they can all too easily switch their appetite off, rather than let normal hunger and a normal appetite for food develop. At its extreme, this becomes the slimmers' disease, anorexia nervosa. The reverse – thinking you are of normal weight when you are overweight – is, if anything, a rarity. Most of us *know* when we are overweight.

Unfortunately, there are no magic diets, vitamins or minerals that will switch your appetite on or off as necessary. Slimming drugs do help suppress the appetite and can be quite successful in assisting short-term weight loss. The tremendous disadvantage is, however, that when the drugs are stopped, the amount of weight regained is almost exactly equal to that lost, and long-term weight loss from short-term use of appetite-suppressant drugs has yet to be demonstrated.

Food craving – the perceived need for sugar

Just as cars need petrol and oil regularly, so our bodies have specific nutritional requirements in order to keep running efficiently. Too little 'nutritional fuel' results in us running out of steam and having difficulty maintaining our body weight. Too much food and drink can leave us feeling wiped out, both physically and mentally. Craving food – particularly chocolate and other sweet food – is very common. Chocolate can in fact provide a temporary 'lift', as it contains theobromine, a chemical known as 'food of the gods', which triggers the release of chemicals in the brain. Chocolate also contains caffeine, which acts as a short-term stimulant. Whilst a 'fix' of chocolate may increase well-being in the short term, this feeling is short-lived, as food rich in refined sugar is metabolised quickly. In fact refined sugar doesn't contain any vitamins or minerals whatsoever, and yet it demands good nutrients in order to be metabolised. The body actually needs foods that will convert into glucose, especially in the premenstrual week when calorie requirements are increased by up to 500 calories per day. Glucose is needed for both normal brain chemical metabolism and nerve function.

Despite the body's actual requirements, food cravings affect approximately three-quarters of all women in the UK, according to our own surveys. We discovered from a survey of 1,000 women with PMS that 80 per cent suffered cravings for sweet food in their premenstrual phase, which led us to undertake a national survey to determine the degree of the problem in general. From the 500 women we questioned in England and Scotland, we discovered that 72 per cent of them chose chocolate above all other sweet food. Seventy-two per cent said they would like to consume fewer foods containing sugar, and just under 40 per cent admitted that weight gain was the worst problem created by their sugar cravings. Twenty-three per cent noticed they became moody and irritable shortly after consuming sugar.

Sugar questionnaire

The following questions relate to your consumption of sugar-containing foods during the last seven days. Before answering them, spend a minute thinking back over the last week and what you have eaten.

During the last seven days:	LOW (none –1)	MEDIUM (2 or 3)	HIGH (4 or more)
How many chocolate bars or portions/servings of chocolate or sweets have you eaten?	1	2	3
How many portions of cakes, desserts or biscuits (1 biscuit counts as ¼ portion) have you eaten?	1	2	3
How many cans or bottles of non-low-calorie soft drinks or servings of ice-cream have you eaten?	1	2	3
How many portions have you eaten/(shop-bought or home-made) of foods containing sugar, e.g. fruit pies, desserts, custard?	1	2	3
How many cups of tea, coffee, chocolate or other drinks *with sugar* did you consume per day?	1	2	3

Total up your score, then ring the grade that applies to you to establish how heavy a sugar-consumer you are.

    0–5 = Low consumer

  6–10 = Moderate consumer

11–15 = High consumer

The mechanisms of food craving

All the New Year's resolutions in the world will not necessarily curb your cravings for sweet food. As firmly as you may resolve to leave sweet foods alone, when you experience the 'munchies', your resistance will be overwhelmed without too much difficulty. But there are good reasons for this mechanism.

The brain and nervous system require a constant supply of beneficial nutrients in order to function normally. Eating nutritious food little and often would probably provide all that is needed, and indeed this is the way we were designed to sustain ourselves. However, our eating habits in the late 1990s are often not sustaining us with enough goodies. Hence the craving for sweet foods can be the body's way of saying that the blood glucose level is low. While a sugary snack may temporarily raise blood sugar levels, it is certainly not the long-term answer, as refined foods soon metabolise and the blood sugar falls rapidly. Nothing short of changed dietary habits and a good vitamin and mineral balance will resolve the problem in the long term. An inadequate diet, as well as large amounts of sugar, can also lead to cravings, which then result in some very unpleasant symptoms. These include:

apprehension	irritability
dizziness	nausea
faintness	nervousness and anxiety
fatigue	palpitations
headaches	sweating

Vital nutrients

Research has shown that magnesium, chromium and B vitamins all have a part to play in normal blood sugar control. Magnesium, as already discussed, is likely to be the most commonly deficient mineral in women of childbearing age, and B vitamins and chromium are also sometimes in short supply. Chromium is interesting, as we are born with only a fraction of an ounce; this is designed to last a lifetime, but inevitably the levels do drop as we get older.

Women who have had several pregnancies and who have breastfed their children are likely to have lower levels of these nutrients, as Mother Nature, in her wisdom, transfers nutrients *from* the mother to ensure that the developing child is well nourished.

Breaking the cycle

The most recent report produced by the Committee on Dietary Reference Values recommends that we cut down on foods or drinks containing sugar by 50 per cent. And since our food-labelling regulations are inadequate, from current labels we are usually unable to determine the quantities of sugar actually present in a product, which makes individual consumption difficult to assess. For example, there are at least 7 or 8 teaspoons of sugar in a can of cola-based drink, and 13 in some brands of ginger beer, and yet there is no requirement for the manufacturers to let the consumer know.

Here are some simple measures to help get you over sugar cravings. (Even premenstrual cravings should disappear within the space of three to four months.)

- Eat regularly. It is important not to skip meals, as this will only serve to make matters worse. If you miss breakfast, your energy levels tend to crash by mid-morning, with symptoms that include a craving for sweet foods.

- Eat little and often. When sugar cravings are severe, it is better to eat smaller, wholesome meals more often, as this helps to balance blood sugar levels. It is worth noting that calorie requirements in menstruating women are increased by up to 500 calories per day in the premenstrual week.

- Cut down on tea, coffee, alcohol and cigarettes. These, along with sugar, serve only to aggravate the cravings, particularly if they are taken in place of a meal, as they cause an increase in the release of insulin.

- Eat wholesome snacks. On hungry days, and in your premenstrual week, have a mid-morning and a mid-afternoon snack. If you are likely to be at work or out and about, ensure you take something suitable with you (see page 157 for suggestions).

- Consume a nutrient-dense diet. Refer to the Nutritional Content of Food Lists that begin on page 336, and ensure that you eat a diet rich in the minerals chromium and magnesium and in B vitamins.

- Take supplements that are also rich in essential nutrients. Over ten years ago at the WNAS we formulated a nutritional supplement containing chromium, magnesium and B vitamins, called Normoglycaemia. We use it routinely as a nutritional prop for the first few months when working

Curbing the Cravings / 93

with a patient to overcome serious cravings. It is taken before lunch (and possibly before dinner in severe cases), as a temporary measure until the diet and exercise take over and blood sugar levels become more constant.

- Deal with stress. If you are feeling stressed or experiencing emotional problems, it is important to address the cause and find solutions. Refer to chapter 12 for some extra help.

- Take regular exercise. This is one factor that can improve the control of blood sugar, as well as having many other health benefits. Exercise increases the sensitivity of the body's response to insulin, leading to smoother control of blood sugar levels. Ideally you should be doing at least four thirty-to forty-minute sessions of exercise per week to the point of breathlessness (see chapter 13).

Chapter 10

What's Your Poison?

Why is it that the things we enjoy most seem to be bad for us? When we are in good health, the general rule is that 'a little of what you fancy does you good'. However, when a personal health crisis appears, it may be necessary to make some sacrifices, and often the very thought of making these changes is worse than actually taking the plunge. Many people feel they couldn't exist without their morning cup of coffee, for instance, but, surprisingly they find the alternatives we suggest relatively acceptable. They actually prefer the health benefits they quickly feel, and are delighted to be free from the 'addiction' or dependency. These latter words may sound strong, but it is not uncommon to find that the withdrawal of regular, but relatively small, amounts of caffeine – one or two mugs of coffee per day, say – can result in withdrawal headaches and other symptoms. Let's look at these social 'poisons' and see just where they fall down.

Caffeine

Many of us have become slowly dependent on caffeine over the years, and our children inevitably follow in our footsteps. Caffeine is found in coffee and tea, but also in chocolate, chocolate drinks, cocoa, cola-based drinks, Lucozade, Lemsip, some painkillers, and the new breed of drinks like Red Bull, Red Kick and Virgin Energy.

Caffeine is one of the substances known as methylxanthines, which act as both physical and mental stimulants. Although small amounts of caffeine can be beneficial in waking us up and stimulating our thought processes, when used in excess it can have numerous adverse effects. Over the years caffeine has been linked to heart disease, high blood pressure and even infertility. We know that caffeine exacerbates nervous tension, anxiety, insomnia and breast tenderness. It can also make you feel restless, nervous, and give you a rapid pulse with palpitations. High caffeine consumers will probably experience withdrawal symptoms when trying to kick the habit, similar to the symptoms produced by alcohol or nicotine withdrawal. If you depend on a caffeine 'buzz', then the road to good health will undoubtedly involve reducing your intake.

Coffee

Coffee is the most widely used drug of our time, and we are consuming more than ever before. Since 1950 the consumption of coffee in the UK, for instance, has increased fourfold. There are many unacknowledged 'addicts' who would find it a challenge to give up, and even forgoing a single cup can produce symptoms of restlessness, nervous tension and headaches.

Ground coffee contains at least 150mg of caffeine per mug, compared to roughly 100mg in instant coffee. When we are well, moderate doses of up to 300mg may be acceptable, but larger doses can produce symptoms that could be mistaken for anxiety neurosis, including headaches, tremors, nausea and diarrhoea.

Weaning yourself off coffee can sometimes be a traumatic experience, but sadly there is no real short-cut. Cutting down gradually over a period of weeks is the best option, and even when going without those extra cups, set aside a couple of days so that you can hide away if you feel really uptight or out of sorts.

How to kick the habit

- Reduce your intake gradually over the space of a week or two.

- Limit yourself to no more than two cups of decaffeinated coffee per day.

- Try some of the alternative drinks, like Barley Cup, dandelion coffee or Bambu, which you can obtain from health-food shops.

- If you enjoy filter coffee, you can still use your filter with decaffeinated versions or with roasted dandelion root, which you can buy from a health-food shop. Simply grind it and put it through a filter, treating it just like ground coffee. It makes a strong 'coffee-like' malted drink.

Tea

The bad news is that tea, the Great British beverage, is not much better for you than coffee. It contains about 100mg of caffeine per mug. However it also contains tannin, another nasty, which inhibits the absorption of some nutrients, zinc and iron in particular. Excesses of tea can produce the same withdrawal symptoms as coffee, but tea can also cause constipation.

Drinking tea with a meal will reduce the absorption of iron

from vegetarian sources by one-third, (whereas a glass of fresh orange juice, rich in vitamin C, would *increase* the iron absorption twofold). Vegetarians and vegans particularly need iron, so drinking anything other than small amounts of weak tea, and that in between meals, may mean that they risk becoming iron-deficient.

ACCEPTABLE ALTERNATIVES – Herbal teas are a good substitute. Unlike conventional Indian or Chinese leaf tea, most of the herbal varieties are free of caffeine and tannin, and they can be both cleansing and relaxing.

A good herbal 'tea look-alike' is Rooibosch Tea, sometimes known as Rooi Tea or Redbush, which looks just like ordinary tea when made with milk. It contains a muscle relaxant, and has been used in trials on babies with colic, and it also has antioxidant properties. Many of our patients at the WNAS prefer it to ordinary tea after a few weeks, but it does take a while to get used to.

There are many delicious varieties of herbal tea, and these days you can buy single sachets to try, which means that you don't get left with a box full of tea you dislike. Our current favourites are Raspberry and Ginseng, Fennel, Lemon Verbena, Lemon and Ginger and Mixed Berry teas.

Caffeinated fizzy drinks

We used to have only cola-based drinks to contend with, but these days there is a new generation of caffeinated drinks to tempt us, such as those mentioned above. Apart from caffeine, there is also the sugar content to consider – approximately eight teaspoons per can of cola – or the chemical substitutes and other additives. Sadly, many young people get hooked on these drinks early on in life, as the 'ad men' would have them believe that such drinks are 'cool' and will enhance their image.

We are all much better off drinking the healthy varieties of fizzy drink, of which Appletise, Ame and Irish Spring are good examples. Or simply dilute some fruit juice with fizzy bottled water.

If you have been a large consumer of the caffeinated varieties of soft drinks, you will have to follow the weaning instructions for coffee. We have had patients who consume 2 litres (3½ pints) or more of cola per day, and their withdrawal symptoms are likely to be quite similar to those of coffee addicts.

Decaffeinated drinks

Decaffeinated drinks usually still contain small amounts of caffeine, as well as other members of the methylxanthine family, and decaffeinated tea also contains tannin. The regulations for decaffeinated cola are that it should contain no more than 125mg of caffeine per litre (1¾ pints).

The decaffeination process uses one of two methods – either water and carbon dioxide, or the Swiss water process (which uses hot water, charcoal and chemical solvents). In the latter process small residues of chemicals remain, but they are minimal. So decaffeinated drinks are better for us but not marvellous. At the WNAS we recommend restricting decaffeinated drinks to no more than two mugs per day.

Alcohol

Whilst small amounts of alcohol on a regular basis do not cause harm, unless you are planning a pregnancy or already pregnant, it is well know that alcohol knocks most nutrients sideways. In excess, it destroys body tissue over the years and can cause, or contribute to, many diseases, among them:

- cardiovascular diseases

- digestive disorders

- inflammation and ulceration of the lining of the digestive tract

- liver disease

- cancer, including breast cancer

- brain degeneration

- miscarriage or damage to unborn children

- osteoporosis (heavy drinking can be a risk factor)

One-third of divorce petitions cite alcohol as a contributory factor. People under stress do sometimes hit the bottle in order to escape from reality, and as most of the above conditions come on gradually, the real dangers of alcohol are often not perceived until it is too late. If your drinking has been escalating slowly, it is advisable to seek help and important to cut your consumption to the recommended limits (see page 328).

Tobacco

Early in the twentieth century cigarettes were actually recommended by doctors, but more recent research has shown that, in all but a few circumstances, they are bad for general health.

In addition, smoking during pregnancy affects the unborn child, and women who smoke more than fifteen cigarettes per day can expect to experience the menopause two years earlier than non-smokers. Smoking also affects bone density, and even stopping smoking at the time of the menopause can reduce the risk of hip fracture by 40 per cent – so it's never too late to stop.

Despite Government health warnings and health-promotion campaigns, people still go on smoking. Research shows that the better-educated have cut back, but younger people, who are perhaps not so well educated, are still puffing away. (Being a parent of teenagers, I know that it is still considered 'cool' to smoke behind the bicycle sheds!) To demonstrate the strong hold that smoking has over us: in 1922 in the UK women aged between twenty and thirty were smoking an average of fifty cigarettes each per year; by 1975 this had risen to an average of just over 3,000 cigarettes per woman, per year.

Giving up

Giving up smoking has never been easy. The first step is to make the decision to quit, knowing that you may well experience withdrawal symptoms, just as drug addicts and alcoholics do when they try to stop. Here is a plan to help you:

- Choose a day on which to give up, and write down the date.

- The day before, smoke as many cigarettes as you can, until you feel sick. Make sure you stub them out in the same dirty ashtray.

- Go to the library and get a book that contains pictures showing the awful health consequences to your lungs of smoking. Look at them from time to time, to remind yourself why you are giving up.

- On the morning of your chosen day, pour yourself a glass of freshly squeezed orange juice, and write down all the reasons for your decision to give up smoking.

- Pin your list of reasons up on the wall so that you can read it at weak moments.

- Put your cigarettes away in a drawer, but tell yourself you can have one whenever you want one.

- When you crave a cigarette, first consider the reasons why you decided to quit. Make a new decision not to light up.

- Go shopping and stock up with some of your favourite wholesome food, including fruit, raw vegetables and dips.

- Tell your close friends and family that you are giving up smoking.

- Take a good multi-vitamin and mineral pill each day, in addition to improving your diet.

- Try to avoid situations that are likely to make you feel like lighting up. For example, drink fruit juice instead of alcohol.

- If possible, go away for a few days to help you break your daily routine.

- Chew some sugar-free gum, rather than eating sweets or chocolate.

- Put the handle of your toothbrush in your mouth whenever you miss your hand-to-mouth habit.

- Each time you feel that you need a cigarette, stop, relax and breathe deeply, so that you get a good supply of oxygen into your lungs.

- Join a gym, and make sure you exercise regularly.

- Don't spend the evenings alone; instead arrange to go to the cinema, bowling or out for a walk.

- If you feel edgy in the evenings, have a few early nights.

- Keep a progress chart, ticking each day that you have remained a non-smoker.

- Save your cigarette money in a jar, and spend it on treats for yourself.

- Practise some formal relaxation, like yoga or meditation.

- If you have a partner, ask for a massage when you feel tense or a bit ratty.

- Picture your lungs recovering now that they are smoke-free.

It is never too late to give up smoking. Whenever you decide to take the plunge, you will be helping yourself to better health *and* preserving yourself for your loved ones. If you find it difficult to quit, contact one of the organisations listed on page 357 and read some of the suggested books on page 353.

Street drugs

These have become increasingly popular in the last fifteen or twenty years. They seem to be readily available and can sometimes be a tempting option for those whose lives are not going as planned. Women of child-bearing age should avoid all street drugs as they undoubtedly harm the unborn child, and in some cases babies are born addicted. Drug users, even more so than smokers, tend to have a less nutritious diet than non-users and are not as concerned about preserving their health, since they are in the process of spoiling it anyway.

Marijuana and cannabis are both widely used substances and products of the hemp plant. The pro-marijuana lobby claims that it is as safe as smoking cigarettes or drinking alcohol. Whilst marijuana does seem to have some medicinal uses, we are not advocating regular use, any more than we are recommending alcohol or tobacco.

Prescribed drugs

At the beginning of the twentieth century, diet and nutrition were used as an integral part of medical treatment. It seems hard to believe that nutrition is no longer considered a major component of conservative medicine, and one wonders how we became such a drug-oriented society. However, with the post-war boom in the pharmaceutical industry, and the power and influence that this industry has been allowed to assume over doctors' education, it is hardly surprising.

In the USA in 1996 nearly $400 billion was spent on medicines by a population of 266 million, and in the UK it was £5.5 billion, or £100 per man, woman and child. Doctors now issue 70 per cent more prescriptions than they did a decade ago. In England alone, over 470 million prescriptions were written in 1995 (nearly 13.2 million for antidepressants), at a cost of £147 million.

Even doctors themselves are now expressing concern about the excessive use of benzodiazepine tranquillisers and sleeping tablets. The current recommendation is that these drugs, which include Valium, Mogadon and Ativan, should be used as a temporary measure for only a few weeks, rather than in the long term. Those who have been taking them for any length of time should, if at all possible, have their dosage and frequency gradually reduced under medical supervision.

When we run into health difficulties, our body depends on us to clean up our act so that the immune system can function properly and do its job. The human body has exceptional natural healing powers, but you wouldn't expect a wound to heal with a nail in it, any more than you can expect to be well without treating your body with respect. So if you currently bombard your body with stimulants, consider cutting down on them, so that your immune system has a fighting chance of keeping you healthy.

Chapter 11

When Supplements are Useful

Few nutritional issues are more hotly debated than whether or not people should take vitamin and mineral supplements. Many experts say no. Many vitamin companies, health-food shop owners and writers on nutrition say yes. The supplement industry is booming in Europe and the USA, while in Australia and New Zealand supplements outsell over-the-counter and prescription drugs.

As is often the case in this sort of dilemma, both sides are right to some degree under certain circumstances. Certainly if you are eating a good diet, not smoking cigarettes, consuming little alcohol, are physically and mentally well, aged between eighteen and sixty-five years and not pregnant or breastfeeding, then you should not necessarily need nutritional supplements. I hope you fall into this category. If you don't, the answer is a definite 'maybe'!

Most common deficiencies

In the UK, according to our own research, the most common deficiencies are of iron and vitamin B and, in women of childbearing age, the mineral magnesium. A mild deficiency detected by blood test may not matter if the diet is essentially well-balanced and the individual is healthy. However, if symptoms or signs of deficiency are present (see pages 56–9), then treatment is required.

A recent survey by the Department of Health of over 2,000 adults in the UK found that iron deficiency is relatively uncommon in men and women after menopausal age. However, 4 per cent of women aged between eighteen and fifty years were anaemic and a further 10 per cent showed evidence of low stores of iron which could not be rectified by diet alone. Often the only clues are mild fatigue and a pale complexion. Any menstruating woman with fatigue should have a simple blood test to check for anaemia. Even treating someone with a borderline iron level can help improve their energy level.

Surveys of UK adults have also shown mild deficiency of one or more of the B group vitamins in 10 per cent or more of the population. This seems particularly likely to occur if you are female, of menstruating age, are depressed or anxious, of limited means or have a poor diet without a regular supply of fresh vegetables, fruit or fortified breakfast cereals. And our own research on women with PMS has shown that between 50 and 80 per cent (depending on the study) have low levels of red-cell magnesium.

So let's now see what a questionnaire to assess your nutrient levels can reveal. Your score will give some idea of your likelihood of having a deficiency of vitamins or minerals. If there is a deficiency, it is important that it is corrected by a good diet and appropriate nutritional supplements. If in doubt, you should of course check with your doctor.

Nutrient levels questionnaire

	YES	NO
Is your complexion very pale?	2	0
If you are a vegetarian or vegan, are you uncertain how to ensure that your balance of different types of protein is adequate?	1	0
Do you have:		
*cracking at the corners of the mouth?	2	0
*cracked or peeling lips?	2	0
*a sore tongue or repeated mouth ulcers?	2	0
*very greasy or dry facial skin?	2	0
On average do you smoke more than 10 cigarettes a day?	1	0
Do you drink more than a total of 8 cups of tea and coffee, ordinary or decaffeinated, per day?	1	0
Do you suffer from anxiety or depression, requiring treatment by your doctor?	2	0
Do you suffer from a poor appetite or feelings of nausea?	1	0
Do you feel tired after little exertion?	1	0
Do you experience mood changes and depression from time to time?	1	0
For women:		
On average, do you drink more than 2 units of alcohol per day?	1	0

Do you suffer from heavy or prolonged periods (7 days or longer)?	1	0
Have you had a baby or been breastfeeding in the last 12 months?	1	0
Do you suffer from period pains or other cramp pains?	1	0
For men: On average do you drink more than 3 units of alcohol per day?	1	0
TOTAL SCORE		

Score:	*Nutritional deficiencies:*
0–3	unlikely
4–6	possible
7 and over	very likely

If you are in doubt about the adequacy of your diet and/or need to lose more than 4.5kg (10 lb) in weight, but are otherwise in good health, you are probably well advised to take a low-dose multi-vitamin and multi-mineral supplement. If you are generally unwell, with any of the above symptoms, you should of course first consult your doctor. Have a good look through the vitamin and mineral charts on pages 56–9 before making any decisions.

It is worth noting that the longer any of the above conditions have been present, and the less well you feel, the more likely you are to have one or more nutritional deficiencies.

Let's now look at some of the different types of nutritional supplements that are available in chemists, health-food shops and supermarkets.

Types of nutritional supplement

Ordinary multi-vitamins

There are many types to choose from. The better ones contain a good range of vitamins and sometimes minerals at a level close to the RDA (recommended daily allowance) or RNI (recommended nutrient intake).

Multi-vitamins and iron

These are similar to the above, but contain additional iron, which is often needed by women with heavy or prolonged periods.

Strong multi-vitamins

These are mainly found in health-food shops and some chemists. They may contain five to thirty times the usual daily amount of some of the B vitamins. These are actually not a bad idea, if you like to down a little more for good measure, or if you experience anxiety or depression. Some may be helpful for particular people, such as Pharmaton for the elderly, and Optivite, a magnesium-rich supplement for women with premenstrual syndrome (available by mail order, see page 360, WNAS).

Vitamins A, C and zinc

Doses of 2–4g per day of vitamin C, 30mg per day of zinc and 25,000 iu (international units) per day of vitamin A (as palmitate) can help to boost the immune system if you are in a low state or suffering from a postviral condition.

Mineral supplements

A variety of mineral supplements are available: iron for heavy periods; zinc to help with acne and poor healing; calcium to help prevent the bone-thinning disease, osteoporosis, though this is best combined with exercise and magnesium. Magnesium can also be used as a laxative, to help premenstrual problems and may be beneficial in some types of fatigue.

Other supplements

There are a number of other scientifically based supplements that are worth a mention, especially as the supplement market tends to be crowded and confusing.

EVENING PRIMROSE OIL – Helpful for eczema, premenstrual breast tenderness and period pain.

MARINE FISH OIL – Liquid, not capsules, which may benefit arthritis and psoriasis. Best taken with other treatments.

EVENING PRIMROSE OIL, MARINE FISH OIL AND CALCIUM – Help reduce calcium loss through the urine and increase the uptake of calcium across the gut wall. These are useful supplements if you are over thirty-five, as your bone mass reaches its peak at about this time, and are particularly useful if you have a family history of osteoporosis.

FOLIC ACID – 400mcg of folic acid should be taken daily by women who are trying to conceive, or who may fall pregnant, from four months before conception right through to the end of the first three months of pregnancy. It has been shown to reduce the risk of birth defects like spina bifida by as much as 70 per cent.

ANTIOXIDANTS – Vitamin A (as beta-carotene), natural vitamin E and vitamin C (with bioflavonoids), and the minerals selenium, zinc, manganese and copper help protect us against cancer, heart disease and degenerative problems, such as arthritis and cataracts.

HERBAL PREPARATIONS – A number of herbal preparations have been shown in clinical trials to be just as effective as drugs in helping to overcome certain symptoms.

Echinacea – A herb that is used to boost the immune system.

Feverfew and ginger – Help to prevent and reduce headaches.

St Johns Wort – (Sold as Jarsin and Kira by Lichtwer Pharma.) The 'sunshine supplement' has been repeatedly shown to help overcome depression, and is more widely prescribed by doctors in Germany than Prozac.

Valerian – (Sold as Valerina by Lichtwer Pharma, Quiet Life by Lane's and Tranquil Night by Blackmore's.) Helps to combat nervous tension and insomnia.

Garlic – Helps to lower cholesterol levels and protects against heart disease.

It is important to remember that there is no special supplement of vitamins, minerals, or anything else for that matter, that will melt your excess weight away. There is no substitute for a well-balanced, carefully selected diet, taking care to ensure an adequate intake of essential nutrients. You will find the foods containing the vital nutrients detailed in the Nutritional Content of Food Lists that begin on page 340.

Chapter 12

Beating Stress

Life in the 'fast lane' inevitably has its drawbacks, and becoming stressed out is one of them. There is a fine line between stress and distress. Stress is reasonably healthy, as it stretches us to capacity and keeps us on our toes. Dealing with challenges as they present themselves is good for our morale, but when we get to the point of overload we cross the line, and our modern-day lifestyle often leaves many of us reeling, feeling overwhelmed and below par. If these symptoms continue for more than a short period of time, our health can suffer.

Beware the warning signals

The rational ones among us do not usually take on a complete 'case load' all at once; we don't ask to be overwhelmed, it just happens to us. We collect our responsibilities as we go along. Perhaps we have been coasting along quite successfully, then a promotion comes along, which demands more from us, and at the same time a close relative gets sick or our partner gets made redundant, then we find we are pregnant again, and so on. Additionally, when asked to commit to a project, some of us have not learned to say 'no'. So we soldier on, believing that we can manage somehow, until one day our body sends out a warning. Whilst this scenario is occurring we are probably snacking instead of eating properly, and not doing much in the way of exercise or relaxation.

The first warning might be a bout of flu, or the onset of headaches, as the stresses of life place extra strain on our immune system; they may also affect our digestive system or energy levels. Were we to re-evaluate our runaway lifestyle at this point, and invest time in getting our body back into shape, we might well be able to circumvent the health crisis brewing. Invariably, though, we get up from our sick bed and step into the ring for the next round. Many of us feel that we have to cope, no matter what, as there does not seem to be an alternative. Women are particularly prone to this form of martyrdom. And it is a vicious circle: because we feel so awful, ordinary tasks become more demanding, and looking after ourselves is the last thing we have time to consider. We may not necessarily have a nervous breakdown, but we can develop a weakness in some area of our body as a result of an immune-system dysfunction. Some of us develop migraine headaches; others get recurrent thrush, irritable bowel syndrome, panic attacks, depression, chronic fatigue or a nervous rash. The unlucky minority will develop a really serious medical condition or have a fatal heart attack.

Whilst all this has been going on, it is likely that many of us will have become regular visitors to our doctor's surgery, and will have begun taking the 'appropriate' medication. So we are now treating the symptoms, and at best suppressing them. You might even get labelled 'neurotic' if you are really persistent.

What we actually should be doing at this point is looking seriously for the root cause of the problem and then addressing it. Whilst some doctors are enlightened and may question you about your troubles or refer you for counselling, they are used to dishing out 'a pill for an ill'. They usually do not have time in their short consultation to find out what really underlies your symptoms. (At the WNAS we take a whole hour for our first consultation and have to be organised about using the time wisely, in order to get the measure of the actual problem.)

Many of us have the ability to cope with near-tragedy or disaster, and it is not until it is over, and the dust has settled, that we feel it is safe to 'fall apart'. With hindsight, the warning signals were all there and we could have avoided the situation, had we come to our senses soon enough.

There is plenty of medical evidence to support the fact that persistent stress (or distress) can affect us both physically and mentally. Let's look at some of the ways you can help yourself before you get really sick.

Tips on handling stress

Here are some tips to help you cope next time you feel under enormous pressure or experience a symptom that may be a warning signal!

- Make sure you have some sacred time to yourself: time to think, and time to switch off from your responsibilities.

- Tell your family how you feel, and ask for their support whilst you get yourself sorted out.

- If your stress comes from work, discuss with colleagues how you can make changes; or if you are self-employed, you will need to re-evaluate your working situation and conditions.

- Try to get away, even if it's only for a few days. Sometimes we can see things more clearly from a distance.

- Learn not to take on too much – if you feel fully committed, learn to say 'no'.

- Prioritise your responsibilities and see if you can off-load or delegate some of the less important tasks.

- Eat regular, wholesome meals and have a supply of nutritious snacks at hand. Don't fall into the trap of missing meals and eating junk food or chocolate instead.

- Take time each week to exercise – you should be doing at least three or four thirty-or forty-minute sessions of exercise per week, even if it's just skipping or a work-out to a video at home.

- Make time each day to relax formally – you will need fifteen minutes, with no interruptions. Really switching off is an art, and you may need some instruction or to read a book on the subject.

- Get your partner or a close friend to give you a massage, preferably using some relaxing aromatherapy oils, like geranium or lavender.

- Watch an entertaining film or make time to read a good book.

- Make sure you laugh occasionally. Laughter is so good for us, and yet when we get absorbed with the problems in our lives we seem to lose our sense of humour.

- Sing in the bath! This has been shown to influence our brain chemistry positively, putting us in a happier and more relaxed frame of mind.

- Pay a visit to a good acupuncture clinic: a few sessions are likely to help you to feel stronger and more able to cope.

- Take some herbal tranquillisers to help you to relax and to put things in perspective, such as Lane's Quiet Life, Valerina by Lichtwer Pharma or Tranquil Night by Blackmore's. All of these are effective, but not addictive, and they do not have the side-effects of drugs.

- If you can't see a solution to your current stresses, find someone to talk it through with, or get professional help. Most GP practices have counsellors attached to them, so don't be afraid to ask for help.

Chapter 13

Waking Up to Exercise

The positive value of exercise should never be underestimated. At this point the non-exercisers among us are probably groaning, but they should sit up and take note. For regular exercise is of great benefit to people of all ages, because it is necessary for the optimum function, structure and preservation of muscles, bones, joints and heart. Not only does exercise give us the feel-good factor on the day, but it can also improve the quality and length of our active life. Regular exercise helps to prevent debilitating and often fatal conditions like heart disease and the crippling, bone-thinning disease osteoporosis, and reduces our risk of having a stroke. Women in particular are more prone to these life-shattering conditions after the menopause, and it's never too early to start preventing them.

Exercise also helps to keep skin looking healthy, as it promotes circulation; and the increased energy expenditure has a direct relationship to the amount of weight an overweight person is likely to lose. For although obesity is associated with raised blood cholesterol, heart disease and high blood pressure, vigorous exercise reduces the risk of an overweight person contracting one of these conditions to almost the same level as that of a non-overweight person.

The energy used while exercising burns additional calories and therefore helps to increase your resting metabolic rate – or the rate at which energy is used up. Providing you stick to the recommended diet and don't start consuming lots of additional calories, you get into what is known as calorie deficit. This means that if you do an hour's vigorous exercise instead of sitting in a chair for an hour, you could burn up an extra 100–200 calories, which would otherwise have contributed to your waistline.

How much exercise is needed?

At the WNAS, we encourage our patients to exercise to the point of breathlessness, in order to increase their cardiac output and trigger the release of the brain chemicals known as endorphins. Whilst a regular exerciser may need to do a full hour of vigorous exercise in order to achieve this, a non-exerciser may need to do only a few minutes initially, until they have built up their stamina. Physical exercise is an important factor in maintaining fitness and energy balance, but you do need to begin exercising at the correct pace. If the programme you choose is too vigorous initially, it will only leave you feeling achy, tired and dispirited. If, on the other hand, your exercises are insufficient to stimulate your limb and heart muscles, so providing aerobic benefit, you will be effectively wasting your time.

Many of us associate aerobic exercise with the local gym or an hour's keep-fit class, and whilst these activities will achieve increased cardiac output, there are many other activities that will do just as well. Brisk walking, swimming, skipping, cycling, jogging and even disco-dancing, for example, are all aerobic exercises. Aerobic exercise is any exercise that stimulates the large groups of muscles in your body, thereby increasing oxygen intake. Over a period of time, these muscles – including the heart, which is a muscular organ – become more efficient.

Eventually the heart can work more slowly, but with increased capability. Once you have achieved increased cardiac function, you will usually experience a greater sense of well-being, on both a physical and mental level, and will be less likely to have heart problems later in life, if you maintain your exercise routine.

In order to protect your health, and reap the on-going benefits that aerobic exercise can provide, you have to continue to exercise regularly, ideally for at least thirty to forty minutes, three or four times per week.

Choosing an exercise plan

Unless you are an established exerciser, you need to find out how to make a start by answering the following questionnaire.

Exercise questionnaire

Tick any answer that applies to you now	Score
Are you grade 3 obese? (See the height/weight chart on page 00)	3
Are you grade 2 overweight?	2
Are you grade 1 overweight?	1
Do you currently do no exercise whatsoever?	3
Do you currently do some gentle exercise occasionally?	2
Do you exercise once or twice per week in a formal setting?	1
Do you exercise more than three times per week for more than half an hour each time?	0

| Do you get puffed out easily? | 2 |

| Can you run up and down the stairs without panting? | 0 |

Which of the following best describes you:
• very unfit	3
• unfit	3
• not as fit as you should be	2
• moderately fit	1
• fit	0
• in excellent physical condition!	0

If you scored 0   You don't need any help with exercise, you are doing just fine.

4 or under   You are not doing too badly, but there is certainly room for improvement. Follow the instructions for moderately overweight.

5 plus   There is plenty of work to be done. Follow the instructions for overweight and unfit.

VERY OVERWEIGHT AND UNFIT – If you are very overweight (grade 3, see page 82) and get puffed out easily, do little or no exercise and consider yourself unfit, you should begin by following the recommendations gradually, after checking with your doctor. Start by exercising gently for five to ten minutes per day, and build up gradually over a period of a month. Walking and swimming are good stamina-building exercises.

MODERATELY OVERWEIGHT AND NOT AS FIT AS YOU SHOULD BE – If you are moderately overweight (grades 1 or 2, see page 82) and get puffed easily, do little or no exercise and consider yourself unfit, you too should begin by exercising gently. If you are reasonably fit to start with, you will be able to increase your pace that much faster. Begin by going for a walk each day for half an hour or so. Gradually increase your pace to the point where you are walking briskly and up can feel your heart pumping away efficiently, but not to the point where you feel at all overwhelmed. A good way to tell whether you are overdoing it is that you should still be able to talk whilst you are exercising.

MILDLY OVERWEIGHT AND EXERCISE OCCASIONALLY – If you are a little overweight for your height (grade 1, see page 82) and are doing some moderate exercise each week, but feel that it's not really enough and that you could be doing a lot better, you need to follow an 'improver' programme. This will involve stepping up your pace gradually, and increasing the number of times you exercise each week. Swimming or aqua-fit are two good methods of exercise that get all your muscles working without experiencing the 'after aches', post-exercise muscle strain.

OVERWEIGHT BUT FIT – If you are overweight, but are exercising happily at least four times per week, then far be it from me to interfere. Continue with your routine whilst you follow the diet.

Enjoying your exercise time

The secret to sustaining your exercise programme is to select the kind of exercise you actually enjoy. If 'enjoyment' is not a term you have ever used to describe your time exercising, then you need to get yourself into the right frame of mind. Unless you come to enjoy the exercise regime you select, there isn't much hope of you sticking to it, is there? Some of us are sporty and others simply aren't. There is little point in arranging to play squash if you really dislike the game, or vowing to go for a jog each day if you hate running. So do select the type of exercise that you could at least *grow* to like.

There is a wide variety of exercise activities to choose from, but remember that the aim is to reach the point of breathlessness. Any one of the following forms of exercise is likely to help you achieve this:

badminton	line-dancing
basketball	rowing
brisk walking	skipping
cycling	sports with children
disco-dancing	squash
exercise class	swimming
exercise routine from a video	trampolining
jogging	

It is probably best to vary the type of exercise you do on different days of the week to prevent boredom setting in. If you have a busy lifestyle it may not be possible for you to get to a specific exercise class each week. And if budget is a factor, then you should look at outdoor activities like walking, jogging and cycling. On bad-weather days I find an exercise video an excellent way to begin my day. I particularly like the YMCA videos, as they are broken down into short workable sections and into fitness levels. These can be mail-ordered from the YMCA (see their address on page 360).

Women over the age of thirty-five should be looking at including as many sessions of weight-bearing exercise in their routine as possible, which includes any exercise that involves contact between your feet and the ground. This is a scientifically acknowledged method of generating new bone. Until our mid-thirties, we lose approximately 10 per cent of our bone mass each year, but equally we make a similar amount of new bone, which means the scales remain in balance. In our forties and fifties, however, many of us begin to lose more bone than we make, putting us at higher risk of developing osteoporosis unless we take positive steps to maintain the balance.

If you are not exercising in a class, when you begin your chosen exercise:

- warm up slowly for the first few minutes

- exercise until you reach the point of breathlessness

- then begin the cool-down process

- cool down gradually over a period of a few minutes, rather than stopping vigorous exercise suddenly.

Try to include some exercise into your routine on a daily basis. You will need to specify the amount of exercise you do on the diaries provided in the appendix on pages 335–6. If you are sceptical about sticking to an exercise routine, it may be best to plan out your week's activity in advance in your diary or on a wall chart, and wherever possible arrange to exercise with a friend. Keep the benefits of exercise uppermost in your mind until your regime is firmly established. When you have reached the goal of doing four or so good sessions of exercise per week, work to maintain this, but don't exceed it on a regular basis. Believe it or not, too much exercise can be counter-productive!

Chapter 14

Backtracking to Health

If you set out to read this book merely in order to lose weight, then you have undoubtedly got more than you bargained for. For weight loss alone is an unhealthy pursuit; it should be part of an holistic programme in which you not only maintain weight loss, but also sustain your health and well-being in the long term. It is far better to lose weight gradually, whilst also ensuring you meet your nutrient demands, than to crash diet to your target weight and run the risk of regaining the pounds. Research supports this 100 per cent, as the vast majority of people who embark on a weight-loss diet put the weight back on again.

Mental functions play a substantial role in determining how we perceive ourselves. When we are short of nutrients, our brain chemistry is affected, which subsequently affects thought processes and mood. Putting back into your body what time and nature have taken out is a sound investment. As we are generally living much longer these days (women on average now reach their mid-eighties), it is in our interests to keep our bodies healthy and vital so that we can enjoy the leisure and pleasure years.

To demonstrate further that our nutritional state and lifestyle have a major bearing on our health prospects (quite apart from the influence they have on the unborn child, touched on in chapter 5), research shows that they also have the following benefits (and probably a great deal more besides):

- A high fruit and vegetable fibre diet, which is low in animal fats and rich in vitamins A, C and E (the antioxidants), is associated with reducing the risk of breast cancer by half.

- A diet rich in calcium, magnesium and EFAs, incorporating regular weight-bearing exercise and supplements of evening primrose oil, marine fish oil and calcium, can prevent osteoporosis, and even reverse it in the early stages.

- A diet rich in B vitamins (in particular B_1, B_3, B_6, B_{12} and folic acid), vitamin C, EFAs and magnesium, in addition to taking supplements of the same, can help prevent and treat mental illness like depression, dementia and schizophrenia.

- A diet rich in EFAs and magnesium, with a low animal fat and salt intake, can help reduce hypertension and high blood pressure. In fact, a study of 100,000 nurses with high blood pressure in the USA demonstrated that low magnesium levels were associated with high blood pressure.

- A nutritious diet, particularly one rich in EFAs and magnesium, can also unblock clogged arteries and reduce the risk of strokes.

- B vitamins, the antioxidant vitamins A, C and E, and the minerals chromium, zinc and, once again, the EFAs, have all been shown to help to control diabetes.

In addition, as we have already discovered, taking regular exercise helps to keep us healthy and prevent disease. Relaxation is fundamentally important to many aspects of our health, as well. New research has even discovered that stress hastens brain ageing!

Taking the plunge

We have learned that, at a time when the quality of our food is not as Mother Nature intended, our food choices are all important. The little extra time you spend shopping and planning your nutritious diet will pay dividends in the long term. Your new diet need not be any more expensive than your previous diet. When we worked out what the average premenstrual woman was spending per week on chocolate, for instance, and what is spent on pre-prepared food and alcohol, you may even make savings, especially if you concentrate on buying fruit, salad and vegetables that are in season, rather than making exotic choices.

By now you have the tools to work out your nutritional requirements, and an exercise programme to suit your schedule. Let us now move on to Part Three, so that you can become familiar with the recommended diet plan and get started. You will notice that there are weekly report forms for you to complete, allowing you to make a note of everything that passes your lips, plus details about the exercise you successfully undertake, time spent relaxing, and your supplement intake. Take care to complete these each day, as they will prove to be an excellent reference source as you progress through the three stages of the diet.

The first week of the diet is the hardest to get through, as it is likely that you will experience withdrawal symptoms, especially if you have been a regular caffeine consumer. Don't be put off, but persevere, as any withdrawal symptoms are likely to be short-lived and will be superseded by positive gain. If you do experience moments of weakness, read through the A-Z of Success Stories (see page 9) again to give yourself fresh inspiration.

Here's to a new you!

Part Three

The Plan in Practice

Chapter 15

The Zest for Life Plan – Basic Guidelines

If you have been a yo-yo dieter on and off for years, the thought of starting yet another diet may give you that *déjà vu* feeling. This experience, however, will be different, for although it may seem unbelievable now, this diet is likely to be the last you will ever need. And not only will The Zest for Life Plan help you shed your unwanted pounds, but you will experience a 'side-effect' of increased health and well-being. There are untold health benefits, both short- and long-term, as a result of following the plan carefully over a period of several months. After the initial loss of fluid, which can be a lot in the first month, you are aiming for steady, gradual weight loss, rather than anything dramatic.

The aims of ZFL

As well as promoting weight loss (if that is your objective), The Zest for Life Plan has been designed to fulfil a number of important criteria. It is:

- a balanced diet that will provide you with all the basic proteins, carbohydrates, beneficial fats, vitamins and minerals that your body actually needs to maintain optimum health.

- Rich in vitamins A and C and zinc, which all help to boost the immune system.

- Biased towards foods that contain antioxidants, the vitamins and minerals that keep free radicals at bay, and help to prevent premature ageing and cancer.

- Full of meals that contain a balance of EFAs.

- Laden with food that contains phytoestrols, which are particularly helpful to women, both during their childbearing years and at the time of the menopause.

The Zest for Life Plan is divided into three key stages. Stage 1, which lasts for four weeks, is the cleansing phase; this will help give your body a rest and put back what time and nature have taken out. Stage 2, which lasts for another four weeks, and Stage Three, lasting two weeks, will continue to give you all the nutrients you need, whilst assessing whether your body can currently cope with certain food groups. In essence it is a ten-week plan, which can be extended if you decide it is necessary after reading The Life Plan on page 325.

For each stage there are suggested menus and recipes to follow. As our tastes and lifestyles differ, the plan has been designed to be as accommodating as possible. There are fast-option menus for those who lead busy lives or simply dislike fussy cooking; there are comprehensive lists of suggested breakfasts, lunches, dinners, snacks and beverages for each stage; and there are sample menus for omnivores – those who eat fish and meat – and for vegetarians. Provided you stick to the rules of the particular stage you are following, you can freely pick your menu from any of the sections. For example, one day you may prefer a fast-option meal, another day a vegetarian meal, and perhaps at the weekend, when many of us have extra time to spend in the kitchen, you may go for a more sophisticated menu.

In addition you can refer to the Nutritional Content of Food Lists that begin on page 339 and, with the exception of items that are off the menu of your current stage, you can choose the foods that you would like to include, knowing that they are full of good nutrients. This exercise helps to tailor the eating plan to your individual tastes, making it even more enjoyable.

What about calorie-counting?

You can breathe a sigh of relief, for you are not going to be counting calories, or weighing food. This does not mean that you can eat vast quantities of food at one sitting, especially if you need to lose weight, but instead you can eat slowly until you feel satisfied. This may seem amazing, bearing in mind that most diets do involve calorie-counting, but the thousands of women who have successfully followed the WNAS programme over the years have had neither to weigh their food nor count calories. As I mentioned in Part Two, finding the right plan for each individual seems to have a normalising effect on metabolism, which results in weight loss for the overweight and weight gain for those who are underweight.

Now let's look at the principles of the diet. It is probably similar in many ways to diets you have seen or read about before, but there are some very important differences. There are some further guidelines at the start of the Recipe Round-up.

Stage 1 – the first four weeks

Foods that can be eaten

In the first four weeks of Stage 1, it is very important to eat only the permitted foods. If you introduce other foods you will lose the beneficial effects of the diet and it will be necessary for you to start all over again!

MEAT AND POULTRY – For non-vegetarians, all meat, including lamb, beef, pork, chicken, turkey, other poultry and game, and offal, such as liver, kidneys, sweetbreads and hearts, can be eaten if desired. Meat and poultry can be either fresh or frozen. Meat must be lean, with all visible fat trimmed before cooking. Do not eat the skin of poultry; it should be removed before or after cooking. Try to buy organic or additive-free meat and poultry to avoid antibiotic residues which are harmful to health.

FISH AND SHELLFISH – For non-vegetarians, all types of fish and shellfish are included, which may be fresh or frozen. Do not eat the skin, however, as it is high in fat and calories.

Note – All meat, poultry and fish should be cooked by grilling, dry-roasting, steaming, baking or stir-frying with low-fat ingredients, such as tomatoes or vegetables.

VEGETABLES – You can, and should, eat large amounts of vegetables daily, especially the green variety and salad foods. Ideally, aim to consume a daily salad, and three portions of vegetables. Root vegetables, like potatoes and parsnips, are limited to one small portion per day if desired. Beans and peas, which are protein-rich, are also included in moderate amounts. If possible, use organic vegetables.

VEGETARIAN PROTEINS – For vegetarians and vegans, these are an essential part of the diet. You are allowed all types of nuts, pulses, dried beans, peas, lentils, seeds, corn maize, rice and potatoes, as well as non-fermented soya produce. Vegans in particular should have two or three portions of these per day. Some people experience abdominal bloating and wind with dried beans, which should always be well cooked.

FRUITS – All fruits are allowed, except glacé fruits and tinned fruits in syrup. Keep tinned fruits without sugar and dried fruits to a minimum. If you want to eat bananas (the world's most popular fruit), half a banana is equal to a single fruit portion. Your fruit allowance amounts to three pieces of fruit per day. Fruit can be eaten whole or as a fruit salad.

REDUCED-CALORIE FOODS – Fortunately there are now many excellent reduced-calorie versions of such foods as salad dressings, mayonnaise, soups and baked beans. As a rule, pre-prepared meals should be avoided while on The Zest for Life Plan.

VEGETABLE OILS AND VEGETABLE MAYONNAISE – A small amount of these foods is allowed daily. You can have up to two teaspoons of a low-fat, polyunsaturate-rich margarine, such as Flora Light, per day. There are no fried foods on the diet (you didn't really expect them, did you?), but there are some stir-fry dishes, where you just wipe the inside of the frying pan or wok with a piece of kitchen paper dipped in sunflower or corn oil.

NUTS AND SEEDS – Brazil nuts, almonds, pistachios, cashews, peanuts, sunflower seeds and sesame seeds are very nutritious, but unfortunately high in calories and some people are allergic to peanuts. If you are using ZFL muesli for breakfast, that will be considered your daily allowance of nuts, seeds and dried fruit. The ZFL sprinkle, which is also made of ground nuts and seeds, is allowed on three occasions during the week to help liven up a salad or a fruit dish.

RICE AND OTHER CEREALS – White or brown rice of any variety – long-grain, short-grain or basmati – is allowed. It will often be used instead of potatoes. Rice cakes (rice crispbreads) may also be used in place of bread. Corn and corn products are permissible including crispbreads, pasta, cornflour and polenta. Additionally, buckwheat, sago and tapioca can be used from time to time.

BREAKFAST CEREALS – Only cornflakes and rice cereal, and ZFL muesli (see page 195), are included in Stage 1. They contain a useful amount of protein and are often fortified with extra vitamin B and iron. Other breakfast cereals, especially the many sweetened ones, are not permitted as they are high in sugar and, often, fat.

EGGS – Up to seven eggs per week are allowed, unless you are known to have a very high cholesterol level. Eggs are highly nutritious and very good value for money.

Foods to be avoided or severely limited

WHEATS, OATS, BARLEY, RYE, MILLET AND BRAN – All foods made with these are to be avoided. This means no ordinary cakes, biscuits, puddings, pasta, pastry, pies, porridge or breakfast cereals (apart from those mentioned above). There are some cake, biscuit and pudding recipes to be found in the Recipe Round-up. Ordinary bread made with wheat flour is off the menu in Stage 1, but alternatives may be used (see the recipes starting on page 315), but even these should be limited to no more than two slices per day.

DAIRY PRODUCTS – Milk, cream and cheese are also off the menu at this stage. Use soya milk and soya yoghurt or rice milk as substitutes (most supermarkets or health-food shops stock them). Butter or low-fat polyunsaturated spreads are allowed in very small quantities: one or two level teaspoons per day. However, if you suffer from premenstrual tension, painful breasts or a raised blood cholesterol level, you should use a low-fat polyunsaturated spread instead of butter.

Foods containing milk, cream, cheese, milk solids, non-fat milk solids, lactose and the milk proteins, lactalbumin, whey and caseinates, should be avoided. The only exception to this is polyunsaturated margarine, which often contains a very small amount of milk protein, lactalbumin or whey.

Vegetarians (i.e. non-meat or fish eaters) should use soya milk fortified with calcium, and should probably consume either one egg per day or generous portions of dried beans, peas, lentils and some nuts or seeds on most days.

ANIMAL FATS AND SOME VEGETABLE FATS – Animal fats, some vegetable fats, lard, dripping and suet are out, as are palm oil and coconut oil, and all foods containing them. Chemically, these vegetable oils are much more like saturated animal fats than good-quality sunflower or corn oil, which are high in healthier polyunsaturates. Hard margarines, which are made from hydrogenated vegetable oils, are also off the menu.

SUGAR, HONEY, GLUCOSE AND FRUCTOSE (FRUIT SUGAR) – Any food made with these should in the main be avoided. This means cakes, biscuits, most ice-cream, sweets of all kinds, chocolate and puddings. This is not as depressing as it sounds. You will find many suggestions for low-calorie desserts during the diet.

Fruit juices are high in fructose, which weight for weight

contains the same number of calories as sucrose (ordinary table sugar). If you wish to include fruit juice in your diet on a regular basis, water it down. And leave large helpings of honey to the bees!

ALCOHOLIC BEVERAGES – You name it – alcohol is initially out. Sorry! Don't do this diet over Christmas. Even low-calorie alcoholic drinks – though they are a great improvement – are too high in calories. You will, however, get the chance to reintroduce alcohol in the long-term plan.

YEAST-RICH FOODS – This includes any foods containing yeast extract, such as Marmite, Bovril, Oxo, Knorr and other stock cubes, vinegar, pickled food, chutneys, piccalilli, sauces and condiments containing yeast extract or vinegar.

SALT – Salt should not be used in cooking or at the table. This is particularly true if you experience fluid retention or high blood pressure. Salty meats such as ham and bacon should be eaten sparingly. Crisps, peanuts and many convenience meals are not on the menu at all. If you really cannot do without, use a very small amount only (natural rock or sea salt) or, better still, a potassium-rich salt substitute like LoSalt. Try flavouring salads, vegetables or cooked main dishes with pepper or herbs instead of salt. You should find that your need for salt becomes less as you progress through the diet.

CAFFEINE AND TANNIN – Both caffeine and tannin should be kept to an absolute minimum, or better still, substituted with alternative drinks. You may recall that caffeine can be found in coffee, tea, chocolate and cola, plus some over-the-counter drugs. Tannin is usually found in tea and red wine. Try to have no more than two decaffeinated drinks per day, as even these contain other chemicals. Instead use alternatives like dandelion coffee (particularly ground dandelion root rather than instant), Rooibosch Tea, which is a good tea 'look-alike', chicory or any of the herbal teas.

FOODS CONTAINING ADDITIVES – Additives cannot be avoided completely, but it is best to avoid those foods with certain types of colourings and preservatives that can cause asthma, nettle rash (urticaria), eczema and possibly migraine.

Whenever possible, avoid the following additives.

E102   Tartrazine

E104   Quinoline Yellow

E110   Sunset Yellow FCF or Orange Yellow

E122   Carmoisine or Azorubine

E123   Amaranth

E124   Ponceau 4R or Cochineal Red A

E127   Erythrosine BS

E131   Patent Blue V

E132   Indigo Carmine or Indigotine

E142   Green S or Acid Brilliant

E142   Green BS or Lissamine Green

E151   Black PN or Brilliant Black PN

E180   Pigment Rubine or Lithol Rubine BK

E220   Sulphites (these may worsen asthma in very sensitive
–227   individuals).

Other colourings are not likely to cause adverse reactions.

SUSPECT FOODS – Avoid any foods that you know do not suit you. Many people, for example, find some fruits, such as oranges or pineapple, too acidic. A not infrequent problem is the inability to digest beans, peas and some vegetables properly, resulting in excessive wind. Possible offending vegetables include cabbage, cauliflower, onions, leeks, green peppers and sweet-corn. At this point, trust your own knowledge and experience. After all, it is this that you want to increase, so don't contradict anything you already know. You may have to adapt the day's menu or recipes accordingly.

Symptoms

You may notice during the beginning of Stage 1 that you experience some withdrawal symptoms as a direct result of giving up certain foods and drinks that you usually consume. These symptoms may range from headaches to fatigue or even depression. The degree to which you suffer will depend on your existing diet. For example, if you were consuming lots of cups of coffee or tea, cola drinks or refined sweet foods, you may find the first week of the diet quite a challenge! Unfortunately there is no magic button to press that will get you through this phase completely unscathed, but cutting down gradually over a period of days – or even a couple of weeks – does seem to lessen the pain if you have been a heavy consumer of such foods.

It is probably best to begin the diet when you have a quiet week to spare. One word of advice to women of childbearing age is to begin the diet just after your period has arrived and not in the week when it is due. You want to prevent additional symptoms occurring at a time when you might be suffering from PMS.

You will need time to accustom yourself to your new way of eating, and require plenty of relaxation. This doesn't mean that you should take time off work; quite the opposite, as it is preferable that you remain occupied while on the diet. Just keep social arrangements that involve eating to a minimum. Then, if you feel tired or experience any withdrawal symptoms, you can go off to rest without any guilty feelings about having let others down.

After the first week or so of following the diet, with any possible withdrawal symptoms behind you, things should look up. By Week 3, you should have lost a few pounds – at least 4 lb, possibly as many as 8 lb (1.8–3.6kg) – and you may notice that a number of minor health problems have begun to improve. By Week 4, you should be feeling quite well, perhaps better than you have felt for some time and, with any luck, you will be a good deal nearer your target weight. It is important to continue with Stage 1 until any symptoms you have been suffering, like fatigue, anxiety, bowel problems or headaches, have abated. This will allow you to attribute any symptoms you experience in Stages 2 or 3 to the foods you then introduce, rather than to any chronic health problem.

Stage 2 – The second four weeks

During this phase you will be introducing new foods in rotation to see whether they are currently acceptable or not. Once you have cleared your system during Stage 1, you should find that your body becomes amazingly good at helping you to identify the things it likes and dislikes. It communicates via signs and symptoms, thus allowing you to become a 'nutritional detective'. Very often, when the immune system is impaired and the body reacts to certain foods or drinks, the chemicals produced may make you feel unwell in some way. The symptoms may vary from a headache, even a full-blown migraine, to eczema, nettle rash (urticaria), rhinitis, asthma, abdominal bloating and discomfort, constipation, diarrhoea, wind, anxiety, irritability, insomnia and possibly PMS, panic attacks or feelings of total exhaustion. The reaction may even push your weight back up, which gives you an instant clue that all is not well.

You will see from the sample menus for Stage 2 that we are about to reintroduce oats, barley, rye and dairy produce (milk, cheese, yoghurt and butter) over the course of the next four weeks. The method of introduction is rather crucial, however. You need to introduce *one* type of food at a time over a period of a few days, to enable your body to report back to you. If you introduce several foods in quick succession, you will only end up getting confused and having to begin the process again.

I have started by introducing oats to the menus, but this is optional; you may prefer to first introduce something else that you have been missing. I have introduced dairy products: first milk on Day 1, then yoghurt on Day 5, followed by cheese. Towards the end of the two weeks' sample menus I have introduced rye. I have squeezed the new foods into my two weeks' sample menus, but you have four weeks in which to introduce them, so it is important not to rush. As a general rule, at the WNAS we allow five days between the introduction of new foods, giving the body plenty of time to respond, if it is going to.

If, and when, you do have a reaction to individual food groups, you may feel that you have had a setback. On the contrary, any reaction should be regarded as a positive step. It means that you have discovered some foods that don't really suit your body at the moment. A reaction may range from mild to severe, but is not likely to last for more than a few days, gradually wearing off. If you do experience a reaction, you will need to stop eating the suspect foods; further instructions can be found in Stage 1.

Weekly diaries

Diaries are provided in the Appendices, which will give you the opportunity to record all foods, drinks and supplements that pass your lips each day, as well as any exercise and relaxation that you undertake. In addition, you have space in the diaries to record any symptoms you experience, ranging from withdrawal symptoms to food and drinks in the first few weeks of the plan to adverse symptoms you may experience when introducing new food groups to your regime as you progress. Whilst the prospect of daily administration may seem like hard work, research over a number of years has shown that the effort will pay dividends. The prospect of maintaining a daily diary will undoubtedly encourage you to follow the rules to the letter, and even go the extra mile as far as exercise and relaxation are concerned, perhaps at a time when you would otherwise turn over and go back to sleep. Once you have established your programme, and begin to experience the benefits, it will become easier. The records become increasingly important in Stages 2 and 3, when reintroducing foods and drinks that have been omitted from your diet for several weeks. They provide an on-going picture, essential to the efficient monitoring of your progress.

Stage 3 – The final two weeks

During this two-week stage, you will be reintroducing wheat, but only white flour products, which contain less gluten and phytic acid than their whole wheat counterparts. We very often find that white flour products, like bread, pasta, pastry and pizza base, are more easily tolerated by the body and are less likely to cause a chemical antibody reaction. Whole wheat products are reserved for trial in the long term, as you will see from the Life Plan chapter on page 325.

In the menus for Stage 3 I have introduced the different sorts of white flour products gradually. It begins with French bread, as it is even lower in phytic acid and gluten content than conventional white flour products, and is therefore more easily tolerated. You will need to keep careful records during this stage, particularly if weight loss is one of your main objectives, weighing yourself regularly to ensure that the pounds are not returning. If you experience the return of symptoms like abdominal bloating, constipation, lethargy, mood swings, anxiety or insomnia, then it is advisable to stop eating wheat totally for the time being. Many individuals find that, a few months down the line, when the body is in better nutritional shape, the immune system is less likely to react when white flour products are reintroduced. If you turn out to be one of the unlucky ones, then you will have to reserve the reintroduction of wheat products to your long-term plan.

Let's get down to business – it's about time to make a start on Stage 1, but before you do here are some vital tips.

Vital dieting tips

Despite there being no calorie-counting in the diet, there are certain rules that need to be followed in order to achieve success. If you have been battling the bulge for some time, you have no doubt often regarded yourself as your own worst enemy. Equally, you can be your own best friend by treating your eating habits and your lifestyle seriously. With The Zest for Life Plan it is not simply a matter of following a restricted diet; instead you need to learn to pamper your body with the foods it tolerates and likes, whilst working to keep yourself in good physical shape. Your mental attitude and lifestyle are as important as the food selection you take to the supermarket check-out. Initially, as with any new diet, an element of will power is needed in order to keep to the rules, and the following tips will help boost your ability to achieve your goals.

- Make a start on the plan when you have sufficient time to commit to it – ideally when you have a few clear weeks without any major commitments.

- Set aside time for planning, shopping, preparation and consumption of meals.

- Rather than shopping once a week for all your food, it is preferable to shop at least twice each week, especially for fruit, vegetables and salad stuff, as the shelf-life of the vitamins and minerals in them is quite short. Make sure you store fresh produce in the refrigerator or somewhere very cool, to prevent them from spoiling.

- Go shopping before beginning your diet, preferably after you have eaten, so that you are not starving hungry and therefore tempted to cheat. Letting someone loose in a supermarket who is both hungry and overweight should be a criminal offence!

- Make a shopping list as you plan your diet for the week, and take it with you, making sure that you stick to it.

- Eat regular meals, at least three times a day, with two small snacks in between if you feel hungry.

- Never miss a meal, because irregular eating leads to less healthy weight loss and increased feelings of hunger.

- Never eat a meal when you are in a hurry – have a snack instead, until you have time to sit down to a proper meal.

- Eat from a small plate, not a large one: a well-stocked medium-sized lunch or breakfast plate looks more satisfying than a large dinner plate only half-filled.

- Chew your food well and savour each mouthful. Try not to hurry your meals. A good way to break the habit of eating too quickly is to put your knife and fork down after each mouthful.

- Eat fresh foods whenever possible, and if possible prepare just one meal at a time. If this is not practical, try cooking a chicken, for example, to eat cold over a period of several days.

- Grill food rather than fry it, to keep your fat consumption low and to preserve the nutrients.

- Make mealtimes sacred and enjoy your food. First, set aside time for preparing the meal. Always eat sitting down, and only sit down when everything is ready: the meal itself, the drink, cutlery and the required condiments. Do not sit glued to the television whilst you are eating, but instead look at your food and relish it.

Decisions to live by

It is important to identify your personal reasons for wanting to be slimmer and feel healthier. Recent research has shown that people who list the consequences of dieting – both positive and negative – and remind themselves of them regularly during the day do twice as well on their diets as those who just blindly follow routine dietary advice. It is a good idea to write the positive and negative consequence of dieting – both the immediate and the long-term ones – on an index card, which you can then carry around and refer to prior to eating or exercising.

An example of a chart that you could write on an index card, or in your diary, is given below. Give some thought to each column before listing the reasons why you want to lose weight. Complete the chart after eating – not before. Once it is complete, refer to it at mealtimes, and any time when you feel tempted to cheat!

Immediate consequences

Following The Zest for Life Plan

a) Positive

Improved mood – Feeling of well-being – Self-satisfaction – Approval from friends and family – Weight loss.

b) Negative

Bother of educating oneself – Possible withdrawal symptoms – Changing old habits – Having to change lifestyle – Changing family eating habits – Having to exercise.

Continuing with previous eating habits

a) Positive

No changes required – Short-term satisfaction – No expense on new clothes.

b) Negative

Poor self-image – Feel bloated and overweight – Feel generally below par.

Long-term consequences

Following The Zest for Life Plan

a) Positive

Feeling of well-being – Pleasing appearance – Sense of achievement –Improved health for all the family.

b) Negative

Unable to indulge in favourite foods and drinks.

Continuing with previous eating habits

a) Positive

No effort required – Social satisfaction of 'free' eating.

b) Negative

Self-conscious of size – Feel uncomfortable and bloated – Feel unwell – Increased health risks – Expense of buying larger-clothes!

Having digested all the rules, you are now ready to set out on your voyage through Stage 1.

Chapter 16

Stage 1 – Foods and Menus

In the next three sections, I give a listing of all the foods, recipes and ideas that are suitable for each individual stage. Here we have Stage 1, which is the cleansing phase of the plan, so the recommendations should be followed very carefully.

A star beside a suggestion means that there is a recipe in the Recipe Round-up; a **V** means that the food or recipe is suitable for vegetarians.

Note that 'alternative crackers' means rice cakes, corn crispbreads or Glutano crackers, available from health food shops. 'Alternative bread/toast/soldiers' means using home-made or shop-bought bread that is free from wheat, oats, barley, rye, millet and bran.

Breakfasts

- **V** ZFL muesli*
- **V** Fruit salad with ZFL sprinkle*
- **V** Corn and rice pancakes* with stewed fruit filling
- **V** Puffed rice with chopped fresh fruit
- **V** Cornflakes with fresh fruit and chopped nuts
- **V** Boiled egg with rice cakes/corn crispbread, or alternative soldiers
- **V** Scrambled eggs, mushrooms and tomatoes with rice cakes/corn crispbreads or alternative soldiers
- **V** Poached eggs, alternative toast and sugar-free marmalade or conserve

- **V** Soya yoghurt, chopped nuts and fresh fruit
- Poached haddock or cod with grilled tomatoes
- and mushrooms
- **V** Alternative toast and organic nut butter

With cereal or muesli have either soya milk, soya yoghurt or rice milk.

Lunches

Select a salad from the salad options starting on page 271 to have with any of the following soups or fast options.

Soups

Any home-made soup or nearly 'home-made' soup like the Covent Garden range (without modified starch). Here are a few suggestions:

- **V** Bean and carrot soup*
- **V** Brown lentil soup*
- **V** Orange and carrot soup*

Fast Options

- **V** Beans on alternative toast*
- **V** Brown lentil Scotch eggs*
- Chicken drumstick
- Cold meat and salad
- Grilled herring, mackerel or sardines
- **V** Herb tofu*
- **V** Hummus with crudités,
- and corn wafers
- **V** Jacket potato with baked beans
- **V** Mixed bean salad
- **V** Omelette
- Potato and herb omelette*
- **V** Rice salad with nuts
- **V** Stir-fry vegetables and rice
- Tinned mackerel and salad

- Turkey breast
- **V** Vegetable and dhal jackets*

- **V** Vegetarian pâté and crudités with corn crispbreads or rice cakes

Dinners

- Almond trout*
- Chicken paprika*
- Chicken with almonds*
- Chicken with peach sauce*
- Cumin chicken*
- Fish stew with peppers*
- Haddock Florentine*
- Haddock parcels*
- Halibut fruit*
- Hot fruity chicken*
- Japanese sardines*
- Lamb and apricot pilaff*
- Lamb and aubergine bake*
- Lamb and parsley stew*

- Liver with orange*
- Mackerel with lemon stuffing*
- Poached halibut with parsley sauce*
- Prawn and vegetable stir-fry*
- Salmon steaks with ginger*
- Spicy fish*
- Stuffed mackerel*
- Sussex casserole*
- Turkey and chickpeas with rice*
- Winter chicken*

Fast Options

- **V** Broccoli and cauliflower in a white sauce (made with cornflour) and jacket potato
- Cold meat or fish salad
- **V** Corn pasta with tomato sauce, pine kernels and fresh herbs
- Corn tacos with mince or

beans (**V**), guacamole and salsa
- Grilled gammon with pineapple and vegetables
- Grilled herring with boiled potatoes, broccoli and carrots
- Lamb chops with a selection of vegetables

- **V** Mixed vegetable and almond stir-fry* with rice noodles
- Prawn and egg salad
- Spaghetti bolognaise sauce with corn pasta or rice noodles
- Steak with vegetables or salad

- Steamed salmon with vegetables and rice
- Stir-fry prawns and vegetables with rice
- **V** Stir-fry Quorn with vegetables (or almonds)
- **V** Tofu, bean and herb stir-fry

Vegetarian Options (V)

- Aduki casserole*
- Bean and tomato hotpot*
- Butter bean biryani*
- Mexican omelette*
- Mexican stuffed eggs*
- Mixed vegetable and almond stir-fry*
- Nut and vegetable loaf*

- Nutty Quorn risotto*
- Nutty sprout stir-fry*
- Polenta with grilled vegetables*
- Red lentil and coconut smoothy*
- Spanish rice*
- Vegetable curry*

Desserts (V)

- Apple and passionfruit delight*
- Apple and tofu cheesecake*
- Apple custard*
- Baked apple*
- Banana and tofu cream*
- Corn and rice pancakes*
- Cranberry sorbet*
- Dried fruit compote*
- Fresh fruit salad*

- Fruit snow*
- Gooseberry jelly*
- Jellied grapefruit*
- Orange jelly*
- Peach sundae*
- Pineapple cake*
- Rhubarb and ginger mousse*
- Seed pastry*
- Wheat-free pastry*

Salads (V)

- Bean salad*
- Bean and sweetcorn salad*
- Beansprout salad*
- Beetroot and cabbage salad*
- Cauliflower and carrot salad*
- Courgette and cauliflower salad*
- Fruity cabbage salad*
- Ginger and carrot salad*
- Green salad*
- Minty cabbage salad*
- Oriental rice salad*
- Root salad*
- Spinach salad*
- Summer salad*
- Tomato and celery salad*
- Vegetable salad
- Watercress, fennel and lemon salad*

Dressings

- Orange and herb sauce*
- Spicy lentil dressing*
- Tomato dressing*

Snacks (V)

If you are hungry between meals, especially if you are female and in your premenstrual week, choose one of the following snacks mid-morning and/or mid-afternoon.

- Soya yoghurt and fresh fruit
- Raw vegetables
- Dried fruit
- Small amounts of unsalted nuts and seeds
- Rice cakes, corn crispbreads or Glutano crackers with sugar-free fruit spread
- Fresh fruit
- Japanese rice crackers (ensure they are wheat free)
- Organic corn chips
- Peanut butter with Glutano crackers or ricecakes

Bread Alternatives (V)

- Cornbread*
- Cornmeal muffins*
- Potato farls*
- Potato and rice bread*
- Rice and cornflour crispbread*
- Sussex rice and corn bread*

ZFL Beverages

Hot	Cold
Chicory drink	Carrot and apple juice*
Dandelion coffee (instant or root)	Filtered water
	Fresh fruit juice
Herbal or fruit tea	Freshly prepared
Hot water with a slice of fresh lemon	vegetable/fruit juice
	Miss P's punch*
Rooibosch Tea	Watermelon and ginger juice*
	ZFL fruit shake*
	ZFL milkshake*

Stage 1: Two Weeks' Sample Menus

You can have 1 glass of fruit juice or filtered water with a slice of lemon on waking.

Day 1

BREAKFAST – ZFL muesli* with chopped fresh fruit and soya milk

LUNCH – Turkey breast with oriental rice salad*

DINNER – Stuffed mackerel* with broccoli, mangetout and carrots

DESSERT – Orange jelly*

Day 2

BREAKFAST – Fresh fruit salad with ZFL sprinkle* and soya yoghurt

LUNCH – Grilled sardines with watercress, fennel and lemon salad*

DINNER – Cumin chicken* with brown rice, spinach and cauliflower

DESSERT – Baked apple*

Day 3

BREAKFAST – 1 boiled egg with 2 corn crispbreads or rice cakes with a scraping of polyunsaturated spread on each

LUNCH – Jacket potato with baked beans and green salad*

DINNER – Mixed vegetable and almond stir-fry*

DESSERT – Fruit snow*

Day 4

BREAKFAST – Corn and rice pancakes* with dried fruit compote* filling and soya yoghurt

LUNCH – Nut and vegetable loaf* with courgette and cauliflower salad*

DINNER – Halibut fruit* with braised fennel, mangetout and new potatoes

DESSERT – Banana and tofu cream*

Day 5

BREAKFAST – Puffed rice with chopped fresh fruit and nuts, and soya milk or yoghurt

LUNCH – Bean and carrot soup* with cornbread* and fruity cabbage salad*

DINNER – Salmon steaks with ginger* with onions, peppers and mushrooms, served with rice

DESSERT – Apple and passionfruit delight*

Day 6

BREAKFAST – Two poached eggs with grilled tomatoes, rice cakes and corn crispbreads with a scraping of polyunsaturated spread

LUNCH – Mexican stuffed eggs* with green salad*

DINNER – Polenta with grilled vegetables*

DESSERT – Apple and tofu cheesecake*

Day 7

BREAKFAST – Two slices of alternative toast with organic nut butter

LUNCH – Raw vegetable crudités with corn chips and hummus

DINNER – Hot fruity chicken* with carrots, spinach and jacket potato

DESSERT – Jellied grapefruit*

Day 8

BREAKFAST – Soya yoghurt with chopped almonds, pine nuts, a few raisins and a slice of chopped melon

LUNCH – Chicken drumstick with beetroot and cabbage salad*

DINNER – Japanese sardines* with rice and watercress, fennel and lemon salad*

DESSERT – Gooseberry jelly*

Day 9

BREAKFAST – Cornflakes with a few chopped pecan nuts, a chopped banana and soya milk

LUNCH – Orange and carrot soup* with cornbread* and root salad*

DINNER – Lamb and apricot pilaff* with braised artichoke hearts, green beans and carrots

DESSERT – Cranberry sorbet*

Day 10

BREAKFAST – ZFL fruit shake* blended with 2 tablespoons ZFL sprinkle*

LUNCH – Mushroom omelette with beansprout salad*

DINNER – Nut and vegetable loaf* with braised fennel, celery and mangetouts

DESSERT – Peach sundae*

Day 11

BREAKFAST – ZFL muesli* with chopped fresh fruit and soya yoghurt

LUNCH – Vegetarian pâté and crudités with corn chips

DINNER – Kangaroo steak with jacket potato, baked onions and green salad*

DESSERT – Fresh fruit salad*

Day 12

BREAKFAST – Poached cod with grilled mushrooms and tomatoes

LUNCH – Bean and carrot soup* with summer salad*

DINNER – Haddock Florentine* with jacket potato and carrots

DESSERT – Rhubarb and ginger mousse*

Day 13

BREAKFAST – ZFL muesli* with chopped fresh fruit and soya yoghurt

LUNCH – Jacket potato with tuna filling, and ginger and carrot salad*

DINNER – Mexican stuffed eggs* with sweetcorn, French beans and braised fennel

DESSERT – Apple custard*

Day 14

BREAKFAST – Scrambled eggs with two rice cakes or corn crispbreads

LUNCH – Brown lentil soup* with a stuffed pepper*

DINNER – Almond trout* with mangetout, carrots and cauliflower

DESSERT – Dried fruit compote*

Stage 1: One Week's Sample Vegetarian Menus

Day 1

BREAKFAST – ZFL muesli* with chopped fresh fruit and soya milk

LUNCH – Orange and carrot soup* with cornbread*

DINNER – Nut and vegetable loaf*, with watercress, fennel and lemon salad*

DESSERT – Fruit snow*

Day 2

BREAKFAST – Two slices of alternative toast with organic nut butter

LUNCH – Herb tofu* with tomato and celery salad*

DINNER – Vegetable curry* with rice and spinach

DESSERT – Fresh fruit salad*

Day 3

BREAKFAST – Soya yoghurt with chopped almonds, pine nuts, a few raisins and a slice of chopped melon

LUNCH – Hummus with crudités and corn wafers

DINNER – Mexican omelette* with brown rice and sweetcorn

DESSERT – Gooseberry jelly*

Day 4

BREAKFAST – ZFL fruit shake* with 2 tablespoons ZFL sprinkle* blended in

LUNCH – Bean salad* with jacket potato

DINNER – Polenta with grilled vegetables*

DESSERT – Apple custard*

Day 5

BREAKFAST – Cornflakes with chopped pecan nuts, chopped dried apricots, plus a chopped fresh banana with soya milk

LUNCH – Brown lentil Scotch eggs* with cauliflower and carrot salad*

DINNER – Bean and tomato hotpot* with cauliflower and jacket potato

DESSERT – Jellied grapefruit*

Day 6

BREAKFAST – Boiled egg with grilled tomatoes and mushrooms and two alternative crackers or alternative soldiers

LUNCH – Herb tofu* with green salad*

DINNER – Mixed vegetable and almond stir-fry*

DESSERT – Banana and tofu cream*

Day 7

BREAKFAST – Corn and rice pancakes* with dried fruit compote* filling and soya yoghurt

LUNCH – Beans on alternative toast with green salad*

DINNER – Mexican stuffed eggs* with rice and steamed red peppers

DESSERT – Rhubarb and ginger mousse*

Chapter 17

Stage 2 – Foods and Menus

In this stage semi-skimmed cow's milk is allowed as well as soya milk, yoghurt, rice milk or bio yoghurt. We will be introducing oats mainly at breakfast and lunch-time, and rye after the first two weeks of Stage 2.

Breakfasts

In addition to the Stage 1 breakfasts you can now add cheese and yoghurt plus, after the first two weeks of Stage 2, rye bread and rye crackers.

- **V** Oat crunchy cereal with chopped fruit and nuts
- **V** Oats (soaked overnight) with sliced apple or chopped fresh fruit
- **V** Porridge with stewed fruit compote
- **V** Oatcakes*, rye crispbreads or wheat-free rye bread with sugar-free jam or marmalade as an alternative to rice cakes/corn crispbreads or alternative toast
- **V** ZFL yoghurt shake*

Lunches

Select a salad from the salad options starting on page 271 to have with any of the following soups or fast options – or any of those in Stage 1.

Soups

Choose one of the Stage 1 soups, or one of those below.

- **V** Chilled tomato soup*
- Fish soup*
- **V** Mushroom and mint soup*
- **V** Parsnip and apple soup*

Fast Options

Choose one of the lunch fast options from Stage 1, or the new foods you are now allowed to try, as below.

- **V** Cheese salad e.g. Edam, Cheddar, cottage cheese
- **V** Chickpea dips with crudités*
- Danish open sandwiches with a pumpernickel base and topping of your choice
- **V** Jacket potato with cheese and salad
- **V** Live yoghurt with chopped fresh fruit and nuts
- Omelette with mushrooms and cheese
- Rye bread sandwiches with fish, poultry, cheese or egg
- Salmon scramble*
- Scrambled eggs on rye toast

Dinners

Choose any of the Stage 1 dinners, fast options or vegetarian options, or some of the recipes below.

- Beef stroganoff*
- Frittata*
- Haddock kedgeree*
- Lamb kebabs*
- Lamb in spicy yoghurt sauce*
- Salmon and cheese roll*
- **V** Vegetable loaf with mustard sauce*

Fast Options

- Grilled tuna steak with salad
- V Hard-boiled egg and grated cheese salad
- Kangaroo steak, jacket potato and salad
- Omelette and salad

Vegetarian Options (V)

- Aubergine, tomato and mozzarella gratin*
- Baked nutty onions*
- Cheesy brown rice pie*
- Corn pasta Italiano*
- Mediterranean vegetable and egg grill*
- Oaty chestnut flan*
- Oaty vegetable crumble*
- Root veggie bake*
- Spanish omelette bake*
- Spinach and egg bake*
- Spinach and Gruyère soufflé*
- Mixed vegetable and almond stir-fry* with rice noodles

Desserts (V)

Choose any of the puds in Stage 1, or one of those below.

- Blackberries with hazelnut cheese*
- Country apple pud*
- Grapefruit sorbet*
- Melon ice-cream*
- Passionfruit fool*
- Tropical crumble*
- Yoghurt ice-cream*

Salads (V)

The majority of salads are listed in Stage 1, but there are a few new suggestions below. The dressings are the same as in Stage 1.

- Coleslaw*
- Greek salad*
- Waldorf salad*

Snacks

Any of those listed in Stage 1, including the following.

- **V** Bio yoghurt
- Muesli bars (wheat-free)
- Oat crunchy cereal with yoghurt or milk
- Plain popcorn
- **V** Small amounts of low-fat cheese with wheat-free crackers

Bread alternatives

A couple of new bread recipes/alternatives to add to those of Stage 1.

- **V** Chilli and cheese cornbread*
- **V** Oatcakes* or rye crackers

ZFL Beverages

As with Stage 1, but a few new suggestions.

Hot	Cold
Bambu	ZFL yoghurt shake*
Barley cup	
Caro	

Stage 2: Two Weeks' Sample Menus

Day 1

BREAKFAST – Oat crunchy cereal with chopped fresh fruit and nuts with soya or semi-skimmed milk

LUNCH – Mackerel with watercress, fennel and lemon salad* with an oatcake*

DINNER – Chicken with peach sauce* with rice, braised celery and peas

DESSERT – Country apple pud*

Day 2

BREAKFAST – Oats (soaked overnight) with sliced apple and bio yoghurt

LUNCH – Mushroom and tomato omelette with tomato and celery salad*

DINNER – Salmon steaks with ginger*, mangetout, braised celery and new potatoes

DESSERT – Tropical crumble* and bio yoghurt

Day 3

BREAKFAST – Porridge with dried fruit compote* and semi-skimmed milk

LUNCH – Hummus with vegetable crudités and corn wafers

DINNER – Kangaroo steak with baked nutty onions*, cabbage and new potatoes

DESSERT – Blackberries with hazelnut cheese*

Day 4

BREAKFAST – Three oatcakes* with organic nut butter and a portion of fresh fruit

LUNCH – Parsnip and apple soup* with cornbread*

DINNER – Mackerel with lemon stuffing* with grilled mushrooms, mangetout and carrots

DESSERT – Passionfruit fool*

Day 5

BREAKFAST – ZFL muesli* with chopped fresh fruit and bio yoghurt

LUNCH – Chicken drumstick with fruity cabbage salad*

DINNER – Cauliflower cheese with jacket potato and sweetcorn

DESSERT – Melon ice-cream*

Day 6

BREAKFAST – Oat crunchy cereal with chopped fresh fruit and bio yoghurt

LUNCH – Salmon scramble* with green salad*

DINNER – Beef stroganoff* with braised fennel, carrots and brown rice

DESSERT – Grapefruit sorbet*

Day 7

BREAKFAST – Bio yoghurt, chopped fresh fruit, almonds and pine kernels

LUNCH – Fish soup* with oriental rice salad*

DINNER – Lamb in spicy yoghurt sauce* with leeks, broccoli and jacket potato

Dessert – Dried fruit compote* and bio yoghurt

Day 8

Breakfast – Omelette made with semi-skimmed milk, and a slice of alternative toast

Lunch – Greek salad*

Dinner – Poached halibut with parsley sauce*, carrots, peas and new potatoes

Dessert – Apple custard*

Day 9

Breakfast – Porridge with dried fruit compote* and semi-skimmed milk

Lunch – Cheese with oatcakes* and coleslaw*

Dinner – Chicken with almonds*, cauliflower, broccoli and brown rice

Dessert – Yoghurt ice-cream*

Day 10

Breakfast – ZFL milkshake* with 2 tablespoons of ZFL sprinkle* blended in

Lunch – Grilled sardines with fruity cabbage salad*

Dinner – Salmon and cheese roll* with cabbage, carrots and new potatoes

DESSERT – Corn and rice pancake* with stewed apple and cinnamon filling

Day 11

BREAKFAST – Cornflakes with chopped pecan nuts, a few raisins, a chopped banana and bio yoghurt

LUNCH – Cheese salad with oatcakes*

DINNER – Spinach and egg bake* with jacket potato and sweetcorn

DESSERT – Baked apple*

Day 12

BREAKFAST – Oats (soaked overnight) with chopped pear, sunflower seeds and semi-skimmed milk or yoghurt

LUNCH – Bean and carrot soup* with bean salad*

DINNER – Lamb kebabs* with broccoli, mangetout and brown rice

DESSERT – Orange jelly*

Day 13

BREAKFAST – Boiled eggs with rye bread soldiers

LUNCH – Turkey salad sandwich on rye bread

DINNER – Haddock kedgeree* with mangetout, carrots and brown rice

DESSERT – Fruit snow*

Day 14

BREAKFAST – Rye bread toast with organic nut butter

LUNCH – Prawn salad open sandwich on pumpernickel bread

DINNER – Liver with orange* with spinach, baked onions and new potatoes

DESSERT – Tropical crumble*

Stage 2: One Week's Sample Vegetarian Menus

Day 1

BREAKFAST – Oat crunchy cereal with chopped fresh fruit and bio yoghurt

LUNCH – Parsnip and apple soup* with oatcakes*

DINNER – Red lentil and coconut smoothy* with courgettes, cauliflower and rice noodles

DESSERT – Pineapple cake*

Day 2

BREAKFAST – Three oatcakes* with organic nut butter and a portion of fresh fruit

LUNCH – Cheese with cornbread* and green salad*

DINNER – Aduki casserole* with jacket potato and mangetout

DESSERT – Blackberries with hazelnut cheese*

Day 3

BREAKFAST – Oats (soaked overnight) with chopped pear, pine kernels and semi-skimmed milk

LUNCH – Spinach and avocado salad* with jacket potato

DINNER – Butter bean biryani* with rice, broccoli and carrots

DESSERT – Passionfruit fool*

Day 4

BREAKFAST – Bio yoghurt with chopped fresh fruit salad and ZFL sprinkle*

LUNCH – Bean salad* with jacket potato

DINNER – Nutty sprout stir-fry* with brown rice, broccoli and carrots

DESSERT – Country apple pud*

Day 5

BREAKFAST – ZFL muesli* with chopped fresh fruit and bio yoghurt

LUNCH – Chilled tomato soup* with summer salad*

DINNER – Mediterranean vegetable and egg grill with rice

DESSERT – Melon ice-cream*

Day 6

BREAKFAST – Boiled eggs with rye bread soldiers

LUNCH – Cheese salad sandwich on rye bread

DINNER – Nutty Quorn risotto* with courgettes and spinach

DESSERT – Tropical crumble*

Day 7

BREAKFAST – Two slices rye bread toast with sugar-free jam or marmalade

LUNCH – Grated cheese salad on a pumpernickel open sandwich

DINNER – Spinach and egg bake* with jacket potato, carrots and cauliflower

DESSERT – Grapefruit sorbet*

Chapter 18

Stage 3 – Foods and Menus

In addition to Stage 1 and 2 suggestions on pages 153 and 167, you can now include French bread, white bread and pitta bread, and anything made from white flour like bagels, muffins or croissants. You can now also use plain white flour to make pancakes and sauces, etc.

Breakfasts

Eat anything from Stages 1 and 2, and add in foods made with white flour – French bread makes a good start.

Lunches/Soups

Select a salad from the salad options in Stages 1 and 2 to have with a soup from the same stages.

Fast Options

Remember that, in addition to the Stage 1 and 2 suggestions, you can now add any products that contain white flour, such as white pasta and white pastry.

- Bagels with cold meat or cheese
- Crumpets with cheese
- Filled croissants
- French bread sandwiches
- Pizza with toppings of your choice
- Quiche
- V Vegetable pasties

Dinners

In addition to the Stage 1 and 2 options, pastry, pizza and pasta are allowed back on to the menu, gradually. Follow the instructions on page 148.

- Fish crumble*
- Fish moussaka*
- Steak and mushroom pie*
- Tuna and fennel pasta bake (white pasta)*
- Turkey schnitzel*

Fast Options

As in Stages 1 and 2, but you could add some white bread or toast if you like.

- Fish in breadcrumbs with vegetables or salad
- Flour tortillas with mince or beans (**V**), guacamole and salsa
- Lasagne made with turkey mince
- **V** Pizza (with topping of your choice)
- **V** Quiche and salad
- Spaghetti bolognaise with white pasta
- Stir-fry prawns and vegetables with egg noodles
- **V** White pasta with tomato sauce, pine kernels and fresh herbs

Vegetarian Options (V)

As in Stages 1 and 2, with a few interesting additions.

- Chestnut loaf*
- Falafel with sesame yoghurt dressing*
- Quorn and vegetable pie (with white flour)*
- Roasted vegetable and pasta gratin*
- Spiced lentil cakes*

Desserts (V)

Choose from the vast assortment of recipes in Stages 1 or 2, or try one of the following.

- Apple charlotte*
- Banana cake*
- Lemon fruit roll*
- Pancakes (made with white flour)*

Salads and Dressings

Choose any of those listed in Stages 1 and 2.

Snacks and Bread Alternatives

Anything listed in Stages 1 and 2, plus the few new additions below.

- **V** Crackers and crispbreads made with white flour
- **V** Crumpets or muffins with nut butter or pure fruit spread
- **V** Toast with pure fruit spread/organic nut butter
- **V** Teacakes with a scraping of polyunsaturated margarine
- **V** Hot cross buns/fruit buns

ZFL Beverages

Exactly as in Stages 1 and 2.

Stage 3: Two Weeks' Sample Menus

Day 1

BREAKFAST – Poached eggs on white toast

LUNCH – Slice of pizza and a green salad*

DINNER – Falafel with sesame yoghurt dressing*, pitta bread, and watercress, fennel and lemon salad*

DESSERT – Lemon fruit roll*

Day 2

BREAKFAST – Pancakes* (made with white flour) with stewed apple, sultanas and cinnamon and bio yoghurt

LUNCH – Half bagel with cream cheese and beetroot and cabbage salad*

DINNER – Turkey schnitzel* with peas, cabbage and new potatoes

DESSERT – Dried fruit compote*

Day 3

BREAKFAST – ZFL muesli* with chopped fresh fruit and bio yoghurt

LUNCH – Croissant with melted cheese and Waldorf salad*

DINNER – Steak and mushroom pie* with broccoli, carrots and potatoes

DESSERT – Fresh fruit salad*

Day 4

BREAKFAST – Cornflakes with chopped pecan nuts, a pear and semi-skimmed milk

LUNCH Turkey and salad on French bread

DINNER – Tuna and fennel pasta bake* with courgettes, carrots and sweetcorn

DESSERT – Apple custard*

Day 5

BREAKFAST – Two slices of white toast and organic nut butter

LUNCH – A portion of quiche with watercress, fennel and lemon salad*

DINNER – Fish baked in breadcrumbs with coleslaw* and new potatoes

DESSERT – Fruit snow*

Day 6

BREAKFAST – Oat crunchy cereal with chopped fruit and bio yoghurt

LUNCH – Parsnip and apple soup* with a slice of French bread

DINNER – Pizza with topping of your choice and green salad*

DESSERT – Blackberries with hazelnut cheese*

Day 7

BREAKFAST – White toast with scrambled eggs

LUNCH – Smoked salmon sandwich with coleslaw*

DINNER – Spaghetti bolognaise with a mixed salad and Parmesan cheese

DESSERT – Grapefruit sorbet*

Day 8

BREAKFAST – Bio yoghurt with chopped fresh fruit, pecan nuts and a few raisins

LUNCH – Cheese, turkey and salad toasted sandwich

DINNER – Fish moussaka* with courgettes, carrots and peas

DESSERT – Banana cake*

Day 9

BREAKFAST – ZFL muesli* with chopped fresh fruit and semi-skimmed milk

LUNCH – Orange and carrot soup* with French bread

DINNER – Quorn and vegetable pie* with carrots, courgettes and peas

DESSERT – Melon ice-cream*

Day 10

BREAKFAST – Boiled egg with white toast soldiers

LUNCH – Tuna mayonnaise sandwich with green salad*

DINNER – Steak with cabbage, carrots, baked onions and new potatoes

DESSERT – Pancake* with dried fruit compote*

Day 11

Breakfast – ZFL milkshake* with 2 tablespoons ZFL sprinkle* blended in

Lunch – Greek salad* with pitta bread

Dinner – Fish crumble* with braised fennel, courgettes and grilled mushrooms

Dessert – Jellied grapefruit*

Day 12

Breakfast – Two crumpets with sugar-free fruit spread or compote with a mashed banana

Lunch – Cheese omelette with beansprout salad*

Dinner – Haddock kedgeree* with grilled mushrooms, sweetcorn and mangetout

Dessert – Apple charlotte*

Day 13

Breakfast – Dried fruit compote* with bio yoghurt, and a slice of toast

Lunch – Hummus with mixed salad and pitta bread

Dinner – Hot fruity chicken* with potato wedges, broccoli and sweetcorn

Dessert – Baked apple*

Day 14

BREAKFAST – Fresh fruit salad* with ZFL sprinkle* and bio yoghurt

LUNCH – Vegetable samosa with yoghurt and carrot salad

DINNER – Frittata* with a green salad*

DESSERT – Cranberry sorbet*

Stage 3: One Week's Sample Vegetarian Menus

Day 1

BREAKFAST – Two slices of white toast with organic nut butter

LUNCH – Hummus with pitta bread and a green salad*

DINNER – Cheesy brown rice pie* with spinach

DESSERT – Lemon fruit roll*

Day 2

BREAKFAST – ZFL muesli* with chopped fresh fruit and bio yoghurt

LUNCH – Croissant with melted cheese and Waldorf salad*

DINNER – Mixed vegetable and almond stir-fry* with brown rice

DESSERT – Apple custard*

Day 3

BREAKFAST – Croissant with scrambled egg

LUNCH – Brown lentil soup* with a slice of French bread

DINNER – Roasted vegetable and pasta gratin* with mangetout

DESSERT – Cranberry sorbet*

Day 4

BREAKFAST – Dried fruit compote* with oat crunchy cereal and bio yoghurt

LUNCH – Greek salad* with pitta bread

DINNER – Stuffed pepper* with root salad* and oriental rice salad*

DESSERT – Apple charlotte*

Day 5

BREAKFAST – Cornflakes with chopped pecan nuts, fresh pear and semi-skimmed milk

LUNCH – Cheese and salad on French bread

DINNER – Spiced lentil cakes* with peas, courgettes and new potatoes

DESSERT – Lemon fruit roll* with *fromage frais* or bio yoghurt

Day 6

BREAKFAST – Boiled egg with white toast soldiers

LUNCH – Corn tacos with beans, guacamole and green salad*

DINNER – Chestnut loaf* with broccoli, spinach and brown rice

DESSERT – Pancake* (made with white flour) with stewed apple and cinnamon filling

Day 7

BREAKFAST – Half bagel with tahini spread and a portion of fresh fruit

LUNCH – Mushroom and mint soup* with minty cabbage salad*

DINNER – Pasta with tomato sauce, pine kernels and fresh herbs

DESSERT – Fresh fruit salad*

Long-term snacks

In addition to snacks listed for the three stages of The Zest for Life Plan, you can include some nutritious, but higher calorie snacks (once you have reached your target weight), especially in your premenstrual week.

- Almond macaroons (see Desserts recipes)*
- Cheesejacks*
- Flapjacks (see Desserts recipes)*
- Extra unsalted nuts and dried fruit
- Home-made cakes (see Desserts recipes)*

- Honey and sesame seed squares (see Desserts recipes)*
- Millet and peanut cookies (see Desserts recipes)*
- Walnut bars (see Desserts recipes)*

Use some of the lovely nut butters as spreads and hummus, taramasalata, guacamole or the dip of your choice with your crudités.

Long-term desserts

- Almond cake*
- Apple and cinnamon cake*
- Bara Brith*
- Carrot and date cake*
- Christmas pudding*
- Coconut pyramids*
- Ginger cake*
- Lemon and almond cake*

Chapter 19

Recipe Round-up

The recipes featured in this section have been arranged in alphabetical order, making them easier to find once you have looked them up in the listings in chapters 16, 17 and 18. You will see that each recipe has been coded, allowing you to identify which recipes are suitable for each stage of The Zest for Life Plan.

Suitable for Stage 1 – 1

Suitable for Stage 2 – 12

Suitable for Stage 3 – 123

Long-term only – L

Suitable for all stages – 123L

A Guide to Ingredients

ARTIFICIAL SWEETENER Allowable in moderation. Concentrated apple juice or fructose, fruit sugar, can be used as alternatives.

BAKING POWDER Wheat-free baking powder is available in health-food shops and in many supermarkets. If you can find it in your supermarket, it is likely to be much cheaper.

CHEESE When you reintroduce cheese, use low-fat varieties.

GELATINE Vegetarian gelatine, Gelzone, is available from health-food shops as an alternative to regular gelatine. Either may be served.

MARGARINE Low-fat polyunsaturated spreads are preferable as spreads in very small quantities, and for cooking.

MILK Soya or rice milk is suitable for Stage 1. When reintroducing dairy products in Stage 2 use only skimmed or semi-skimmed milk and preferably the organic variety.

MODIFIED STARCH This is a wheat-based starch unless otherwise stated on the label, i.e. 'modified corn starch'. Until wheat is reintroduced, be careful to read labels in order to avoid starch completely.

SALT Salt and salty food should be avoided, but a salt substitute like LoSalt can be used.

SOYA SAUCE This usually contains wheat, so should be avoided until you are at the point of reintroducing wheat. Instead you can use wheat-free tamari sauce, which is a high-quality version of soya sauce.

Guidelines on Portion Sizes

At the WNAS we do not place a great deal of emphasis on portion sizes, more on the type of food that is consumed. If your main objective is to lose weight, however, it would be preferable to consume medium portions. It is important to feel satisfied by your meals, so chewing food well and eating slowly will help to give you a sense of fullness. As a guideline, a main meal should consist of a portion of protein – poultry, meat, fish or a vegetarian variety – with three portions of vegetables. Together this combination should fill an average-sized dinner plate comfortably, but should not be piled high! Salads can be as large as you like, as they contain very few calories. Nuts and seeds should be consumed in moderation if you are trying to lose weight for, although they are extremely nutritious, they are also calorific.

Breakfast should be a satisfying meal that provides the body with all the essential nutrients it needs to get going efficiently each day. Aim to eat approximately half an average bowlful of muesli, or the equivalent. This measure excludes the fresh fruit, yoghurt or milk that should subsequently be added.

Recipe Flexibility

Once you have become familiar with the Zest for Life Plan you will notice that many of the recipes can easily be adjusted to suit each individual stage. For example, when a recipe contains skimmed milk, soya or rice milk can be used as a substitute. Equally, where plain flour (wheat flour) is mentioned, very often a combination of rice, soya and cornflour can be used instead and vice versa. I am always experimenting with new recipes, so if you devise anything new and delicious during the course of Zest for Life, I would love to hear about it!

Corn and Rice Pancakes 123L *Serves 4*

50g (2 oz) rice flour
50g (2 oz) cornflour
1 small egg
300ml (10 fl oz) soya or rice milk (or skimmed at Stages 2, 3)
a little oil

1   Make a thin batter with the flours, egg and milk.
2   Use kitchen paper to wipe a small non-stick frying pan with a little oil and heat until the oil is smoking.
3   Pour a generous 2 tablespoons of batter into the pan and swirl it around to cover the base. Cook for 60 seconds.
4   Flip it over and cook for a further few seconds. Set aside.
5   Repeat the procedure until you have used up all the batter.

Oatcakes 23L *Makes 12 biscuits*

25g (1 oz) margarine
2 tablespoons water
225g (8 oz) oatmeal
a pinch of salt
¼ teaspoon baking powder

1   Preheat the oven to 190°C/375°F/Gas 5.
2   Melt the margarine in the boiling water in a bowl.
3   Add the remaining ingredients and mix to form a soft dough.

4   Roll out thinly on a floured surface, and cut into 12 portions.
5   Put on to a greased baking tray and bake in the preheated oven for 25 minutes or until lightly coloured. Cool on a wire rack.

ZFL Muesli   123L   *Makes 10–12 servings*

2½ mugs puffed rice
2 mugs cornflakes
½ mug sunflower seeds
½ mug chopped almonds
½ mug pumpkin seeds
½ mug chopped pecan nuts
½ mug pine kernels
⅓ mug organic linseeds
½ mug organic apricots, chopped (optional)
⅔ mug organic raisins (optional)

1   Mix the ingredients together and store in a sealed container.
2   Serve with chopped fresh fruit and the appropriate yoghurt or milk of your stage.

• **Note** If you are constipated you will need to sprinkle an additional 1–2 tablespoons of organic linseeds on to your muesli each morning for the best results!

ZFL Sprinkle 123L

Makes 18 tablespoons (1 level tablespoon = 1 serving)

½ mug almonds
½ mug sunflower seeds
⅓ mug pumpkin seeds
¼ mug golden linseeds

- Use organic seeds where possible.
- Three servings per week are allowed until you have reached your target weight.

1   Grind the ingredients together in a blender to a coarse powder consistency.
2   Store in a sealed container. This gives a new dimension to breakfasts, salads and desserts.

ZFL Yoghurt Shake 23L *Serves 2*

1 large carton bio yoghurt
3 portions fruit of your choice, skinned and cut into segments
ice cubes (optional)

1   Blend the ingredients together in a liquidiser and serve immediately.
2   Blend in 2 tablespoons ZFL sprinkle if using the shake as a meal replacement.

Bean and Carrot Soup   123L   *Serves 4*

1 tablespoon sunflower oil
450g (1 lb) carrots, peeled and sliced
1 large potato, diced
1 medium onion, chopped
900ml (1½ pints) water
1 tablespoon tomato purée
a good pinch of ground coriander
freshly ground black pepper
1 × 415g (15 oz) can kidney beans, drained and rinsed
chopped fresh parsley

1   Heat the oil in a saucepan, add the vegetables and cook, stirring for 5 minutes.
2   Add the water, tomato purée, coriander and pepper to taste, and bring to the boil. Lower the heat, cover and simmer for 45 minutes.
3   Stir in the kidney beans and reheat gently.
4   Pour into individual soup bowls, garnish with parsley and serve at once.

Brown Lentil Soup   123L   *Serves 6–8*

450g (1 lb) brown lentils
1 litre (1¾ pints) water
2 tablespoons sunflower oil
1 large onion, chopped
2 garlic cloves, crushed
1.5 litres (2½ pints) vegetable stock
2 celery sticks, trimmed and chopped
1 large carrot, chopped
1 bay leaf
freshly ground black pepper

1   Place the lentils and water in a pan and bring to the boil. Boil for 2 minutes, then remove from the heat and leave to stand for 2 hours, covered. Drain.

2   Heat the oil in a saucepan and lightly brown the onion. Add the garlic and mix well.

3   Stir in the drained lentils, add the stock and bring to the boil.

4   Add the celery, carrot, bay leaf and pepper. Simmer for 45–60 minutes until the lentils are tender, then remove the bay leaf.

5   Half or all of the soup can be puréed in a blender or food processor.

Chilled Tomato Soup   23L   *Serves 4*

450g (1 lb) tomatoes, skinned, seeded and chopped
100g (4 oz) cucumber, peeled and chopped
1 garlic clove, crushed
a pinch of cayenne pepper
1 teaspoon Worcestershire sauce
1 medium green pepper, cored, seeded and chopped
150g (5 oz) natural yoghurt
chopped fresh parsley

1   Place the tomatoes, cucumber, garlic, cayenne, Worcestershire sauce, half the green pepper and half the yoghurt in a blender or food processor and liquidise until smooth.
2   Chill until cold.
3   Stir in the remaining green pepper and yoghurt, and sprinkle with parsley before serving.

Fish Soup   23L   *Serves 6*

1.8 litres (3 pints) fish stock
4 medium onions, finely chopped
1 medium green pepper, cored, seeded and finely sliced
1 tablespoon paprika
900g (2 lb) filleted white fish, cut into 5cm (2 in) pieces
1 red chilli, seeded and finely chopped
75ml (3 fl oz) fromage frais

1   Bring the fish stock to the boil.

2   Reduce the heat and add the onion, pepper and paprika and stir well.
3   Cover the pan and simmer the mixture for 1 hour, or until the onion is soft.
4   Remove the pan from the heat and strain the mixture. Discard any pulp left in the strainer.
5   Add the fish to the strained stock and bring to the boil.
6   Add the chilli, reduce the heat and simmer for 15–20 minutes or until the fish flakes easily when tested with a fork.
7   Transfer the soup to a warmed tureen. Stir in the *fromage frais* and serve immediately.

Mushroom and Mint Soup   23L   *Serves 4*

4 large potatoes, peeled and coarsely chopped
1 small onion, chopped
900ml (1½ pints) chicken stock
finely grated rind and juice of 1 lemon
1 tablespoon chopped fresh rosemary
freshly ground black pepper to taste
50g (2 oz) margarine
225g (8 oz) mushrooms, sliced
1 tablespoon plain flour
2 tablespoons finely chopped fresh mint
150ml (5 fl oz) semi-skimmed milk

1   Place the potatoes and onion in a large saucepan and add the stock, lemon rind and juice, rosemary and pepper.
2   Bring the mixture to the boil. Reduce the heat and simmer, stirring occasionally, for 25 minutes or until the vegetables are tender.

3 In a small saucepan, melt the margarine over a low heat.
   Add the mushrooms and toss them in the margarine until
   they are thoroughly coated. Cook them slowly, stirring
   occasionally, for 10 minutes.
4 Sprinkle the flour into the mushroom pan and stir it in
   with a wooden spoon. Set aside for the moment.
5 Remove the potatoes and onion from the stock mixture
   with a slotted spoon. Purée them in a blender or food
   processor or push through a sieve with a wooden spoon.
6 Return the purée to the stock mixture. Add the mushrooms.
7 Bring to the boil, stirring occasionally. Stir in the mint.
8 Remove from the heat and stir in the milk. Heat through
   quickly and serve.

Orange and Carrot Soup 123L *Serves 2*

This soup can also be used as a sauce for grilled or roast meats,
or cold as a salad dressing.

285g (10 oz) carrots, chopped
1 medium leek, thinly sliced
350ml (12 fl oz) vegetable stock
a pinch of thyme
75–115ml (3–4 fl oz) orange juice
freshly ground black pepper

1 Place the carrots, leek, vegetable stock and thyme into a
   saucepan, bring to the boil and simmer for 30 minutes.
2 Purée the mixture in a blender or food processor.
3 Return to the saucepan, add the orange juice and season
   with pepper. Heat through very gently.

Parsnip and Apple Soup 23L Serves 6

700g (1½ lb) parsnips, peeled and roughly chopped
1 cooking apple, peeled, cored and roughly chopped
1.2 litres (2 pints) vegetable stock
150ml (5 fl oz) skimmed milk
freshly ground black pepper

1   Put the parsnips and apple into a saucepan and cover with the stock. Bring to the boil, cover, then simmer for 30 minutes or until the parsnips are very soft.
2   Leave the soup to cool slightly then purée in a blender or food processor.
3   Return the soup to the saucepan, add the milk and reheat gently. Season with pepper to taste.

Lunches

If lunch is your lighter meal of the day, it should ideally consist of a salad of your choice plus either some protein – i.e. oily fish, poultry or vegetarian protein like eggs, beans, lentils or seeds – or a jacket potato with a filling, or a bowl of home-made soup. In addition I have included a few slightly more elaborate ideas which might be incorporated into a lunch-time menu if you happen to be entertaining.

Brown Lentil Scotch Eggs   123L   *Serves 4*

1½ tablespoons sunflower oil
2 large onions, finely chopped
1 garlic clove, crushed
175g (6 oz) brown lentils, cooked until tender and drained well
1 tablespoon each of dried oregano and dried basil
1 tablespoon lemon juice
freshly ground black pepper
1 egg, beaten
4 hard-boiled eggs, shelled
1 tablespoon sesame seeds

1   Preheat the oven to 180°C/350°F/Gas 4.
2   Heat half the oil in a frying pan and gently fry the onion for 6–8 minutes until softened.
3   Add the garlic, lentils, oregano, basil, lemon juice and black pepper. Mix well with a fork until the mixture binds together. If necessary, add some of the beaten egg. Divide the mixture into four equal pieces.
4   Dip each hard-boiled egg into the beaten egg mixture and cover with one-quarter of the lentil mixture, squeezing lightly to cover and adhere. Brush again with the beaten egg and roll in the sesame seeds. Repeat this procedure with each egg.
5   Cut four squares of foil, large enough to wrap each egg in. Brush each of these with the remaining oil and wrap each egg. Place on a baking tray and bake in the preheated oven for 15 minutes.
6   Remove the foil carefully, and serve the eggs hot or cold.

Chickpea Dips with Crudités 23L *Serves 8*

2 × 415g (15 oz) cans chickpeas, drained and rinsed
1 garlic clove, crushed
1 tablespoon fresh lemon juice
25ml (1 fl oz) olive oil
175ml (6 fl oz) plain Greek yoghurt
freshly ground black pepper
4 teaspoons freshly chopped parsley
2 teaspoons tomato purée
sprigs of parsley, strips of red pepper and
  pieces of sliced lemon to garnish
To serve
a selection of raw vegetables (peppers, radishes, carrots, celery,
  cucumber)

1 Place the chickpeas in a blender or food processor and blend until smooth.
2 Add the garlic, lemon juice, olive oil and yoghurt and mix well. Add pepper to taste.
3 Transfer one-third of the mixture to a small serving bowl. Divide the rest between two small mixing bowls.
4 Add the chopped parsley to one, stir well and transfer to a small serving bowl.
5 Add the tomato purée to the other, stir well and transfer to a small serving bowl. Adjust seasoning if necessary.
6 Garnish the parsley dip with sprigs of parsley, the tomato dip with red pepper and the plain dip with the pieces of lemon.
7 Chop the raw vegetables into sticks. Arrange on a serving dish around the dips.

Herb Tofu   123L   *Serves 4*

1 dessertspoon vegetable oil
1 small red pepper, cored, seeded and thinly sliced
1 garlic clove, crushed
175g (6 oz) tofu, cubed
½ tablespoon chopped parsley

1   Heat the oil in a frying pan.
2   Add the red pepper and garlic and fry for 2–3 minutes.
3   Add the tofu and parsley and continue to stir-fry until the tofu is heated through. Serve immediately.

Potato and Cheese Bake   23L   *Serves 4*

700g (1½ lb) potatoes, peeled
sunflower oil
2 medium onions, finely chopped
25g (1 oz) cornflour
freshly ground black pepper
½ teaspoon dried mixed herbs
350ml (12 fl oz) milk
225g (8 oz) Cheddar cheese, finely grated

1   Preheat the oven to 180°C/350°F/Gas 4. Grease a medium ovenproof dish with a little oil.
2   Boil and mash the potatoes. Place them in a medium mixing bowl and set aside.
3   Heat 1 tablespoon of the oil and fry the onion until softened and golden. Remove the pan from the heat and

stir in the cornflour, black pepper and herbs to make a smooth paste.

4   Gradually add the milk, stirring continuously to avoid lumps.

5   Return the pan to a low heat, stirring constantly, for 4–5 minutes or until the sauce is smooth and thick.

6   Add 175g (6 oz) of the cheese and cook until it has melted, stirring all the time.

7   Gradually stir the cheese sauce into the mashed potato, beating constantly until the mixture is smooth.

8   Turn the mixture into the prepared dish, smooth the top, and sprinkle with the remaining cheese. Bake in the preheated oven for 25–35 minutes or until the top is golden brown. Serve immediately.

Potato and Herb Omelette   123L   *Serves 4*

450g (1 lb) potatoes, cooked and mashed
3 eggs, separated
2 tablespoons soya or rice milk
1 tablespoon dried mixed herbs
freshly ground black pepper
2 teaspoons sunflower oil
To serve
½ cucumber, sliced
4 small tomatoes, sliced

1   Beat the potato with the egg yolks, soya or rice milk, mixed herbs and pepper to taste.

2   Whisk the egg whites until stiff and fold them into the potato mixture.

3   Heat the oil in a frying pan, add the mixture and cook for 2 minutes on each side.
4   Slide on to a serving plate and cut into quarters. Garnish each portion with slices of cucumber and tomato, and serve with a green salad or vegetables.

Salmon Scramble   23L   *Serves 2*

3 eggs
1 tablespoon skimmed milk
2 teaspoons chopped dill
freshly ground black pepper
75g (3 oz) canned salmon

1   Whisk the eggs and milk with the dill and freshly ground pepper.
2   Cook gently in a non-stick pan, stirring constantly, for 4–5 minutes until firm.
3   Mix in the salmon and serve.

Vegetable and Dhal Jackets   123L   *Serves 4*

2 tablespoons vegetable oil
1 small onion, chopped
1 tablespoon mild curry powder
75g (3 oz) red lentils
75g (3 oz) French beans, trimmed and cut into 2.5cm (1 in)
   lengths
50g (2 oz) raisins

25g (1 oz) desiccated coconut
200ml (7 fl oz) vegetable stock
400g (14 oz) canned chopped tomatoes
4 hot baked potatoes
freshly ground black pepper
toasted flaked coconut to garnish

1   Heat the oil in a saucepan and sauté the onion for 3
    minutes until soft.
2   Add the curry powder and lentils and cook for 5 minutes,
    stirring occasionally.
3   Add the beans, raisins, coconut, stock and tomatoes, cover
    and simmer for 20 minutes, stirring frequently.
4   Cut the tops off the potatoes and scoop out the centres.
    Cut the potato into chunks, add to the vegetable mixture
    and season with black pepper.
5   Spoon a little of the vegetable mixture into the potato skins
    and serve the remainder separately.
6   Garnish with a little toasted coconut.

Vegetable Loaf with Mustard Sauce   23L   *Serves 4*

225g (8 oz) coarsely grated carrot
175g (6 oz) cooked white or brown rice
100g (4 oz) grated potato
100g (4 oz) finely chopped onion
100g (4 oz) chopped celery
75g (3 oz) chopped green pepper
1 teaspoon paprika
2 medium eggs, beaten

Mustard Sauce
25g (1 oz) margarine
25g (1 oz) potato or rice flour
300ml (10 fl oz) skimmed milk
1½ teaspoons made mustard

1   Line a 13 × 20cm (5 × 8 in) baking tin with foil, and preheat the oven to 180°C/350°F/Gas 4.
2   Combine all the ingredients for the loaf in a bowl, then press all the mixture into the lined baking tin.
3   Bake in the preheated oven for 50 minutes and leave to stand whilst making the sauce.
4   Melt the margarine in a saucepan, stir in the flour, and cook for 1–2 minutes, stirring constantly.
5   Slowly add the milk, again stirring all the time over a low heat, until the sauce thickens. Stir in the mustard.
6   Turn the vegetable loaf out on to a plate, and slice. Serve with the mustard sauce.

Dinners

Almond Trout   123L   *Serves 4*

4 trout, cleaned, with heads and tails intact
freshly ground black pepper
juice of 1 lemon
25g (1 oz) margarine
50g (2 oz) flaked almonds
4 sprigs parsley

1   Season the fish with pepper and lemon juice.
2   Melt the margarine and lightly brush over the fish.
3   Place the fish under a hot grill and cook for about 6 minutes on each side or until the fish is cooked through.
4   Brush one side again lightly with melted margarine and arrange the almonds over the fish. Grill again for 1 minute or until the almonds start to brown.
5   Garnish with parsley and serve.

Beef Stroganoff   23L   *Serves 4*

450g (1 lb) fillet of beef, cut into thin strips
2 teaspoons oil
25g (1 oz) butter
1 medium onion, finely sliced
100g (4 oz) red pepper, chopped
½ vegetable stock cube
150ml (5 fl oz) boiling water
1 level teaspoon tomato purée
6 level tablespoons fromage frais
freshly ground black pepper

1   Heat half the oil and half the butter in a non-stick frying pan. Add the onion, and cook over a low heat, stirring frequently, until soft.
2   Stir in the red pepper pieces.
3   Dissolve the stock cube in a cup of the boiling water, stir in the tomato purée, then add to the pan. Boil rapidly until the liquid is reduced to about 4 tablespoons. Tip the reduced liquid into a bowl and set aside.
4   Heat the remaining oil and butter in the pan and add the

meat, which should all fit in the pan easily in a single layer. If necessary, cook it in two batches. Cook over a fairly high heat until the outsides are browned – about 3 minutes each side. Shake and toss the pan frequently as the meat cooks.

5   Add the vegetable mixture and liquid and heat through.

6   Add the *fromage frais* and pepper. Heat through but do not allow to boil.

Chicken Paprika   123L   *Serves 4*

4 × 150g (5 oz) chicken joints
2 teaspoons paprika
160ml (5½ fl oz) vegetable stock
1 onion, finely chopped
freshly ground black pepper
1–2 teaspoons cornflour mixed with a tablespoon of water
1 tablespoon finely chopped parsley

1   Sprinkle the chicken with paprika, and gently grill on both sides for about 5 minutes until brown.

2   Place in a casserole dish with the vegetable stock, onion and freshly ground pepper.

3   Cover and simmer on top of the stove for 30–40 minutes, or until tender.

4   Lift the chicken out of the liquid, place on a warm dish and cover to keep hot.

5   Thicken the liquid with the cornflour mixture. Pour over the chicken and serve, decorated with parsley.

Chicken with Almonds   123L   *Serves 4*

4 chicken breasts
15g (½ oz) polyunsaturated margarine, melted
150ml (5 fl oz) water
a few black peppercorns
75g (3 oz) flaked almonds

1   Preheat the oven to 180°C/350°F/Gas 4.
2   Skin the chicken and brush with the melted margarine.
3   Place the water and peppercorns in an ovenproof dish. Place the chicken in the water and cover with foil. Bake for 15 minutes in the preheated oven.
4   Remove the foil and sprinkle with flaked almonds. Return, uncovered, to the oven for a further 15 minutes, or until the chicken is tender and the almonds have browned.
5   Serve with steamed vegetables, e.g. new potatoes and broccoli.

Chicken with Peach Sauce   123L   *Serves 6*

1.6kg (3½ lb) fresh chicken, skinned and cut into 6 serving
  pieces
freshly ground black pepper
2 tablespoons vegetable oil
1 small onion, finely chopped
1 garlic clove, crushed
¼ teaspoon red pepper flakes
½ teaspoon ground ginger
250ml (8 fl oz) vegetable stock

50ml (2 fl oz) lime juice
50ml (2 fl oz) lemon juice
1 tablespoon sunflower oil
4 fresh peaches, halved, stoned and sliced

1   Preheat the oven to 190°C/375°F/Gas 5.
2   Sprinkle the black pepper over the chicken pieces and set them aside.
3   In a large frying pan heat the oil and add the chicken pieces a few at a time. Fry, turning occasionally, for 8–10 minutes. With a slotted spoon, remove the chicken from the pan and transfer to a medium ovenproof casserole.
4   Add the onion and garlic to the pan and fry them, stirring occasionally, for 5–7 minutes or until the onion is soft and translucent but not brown.
5   Stir in the pepper flakes, ginger and stock, and bring the mixture to the boil, stirring constantly.
6   Remove the pan from the heat and stir in the lime and lemon juices. Pour the mixture over the chicken pieces in the casserole. Set aside.
7   Melt the oil in a clean frying pan and gently fry the peaches for 6 minutes, or until they begin to turn to pulp. Transfer from the pan to the casserole.
8   Cover the casserole and bake in the preheated oven for 1 hour, or until the chicken pieces are tender. Serve with rice.

Cumin Chicken   123L   *Serves 2*

2 × 100g (4 oz) chicken breast fillets, cubed
1 teaspoon vegetable oil
1 teaspoon cumin seeds
½ red pepper, cored, seeded and chopped
3 spring onions, chopped
1 teaspoon finely chopped root ginger
300ml (10 fl oz) chicken or vegetable stock
about 1 teaspoon cornflour, mixed to a paste with a little water

1 Heat oil in saucepan, add the cumin seeds, and stir until they start popping.
2 Add the chicken, pepper, onions and ginger, and stir for 3 minutes.
3 Add the stock, bring to the boil, and simmer for 5 minutes.
4 Add the cornflour mixture and simmer for a further 5 minutes before serving.

Fish Crumble   3L   *Serves 2*

200g (7 oz) cod fillet
1 small onion, sliced
1 carrot, sliced
75g (3 oz) green beans, sliced
3 fresh tomatoes, skinned and sliced
1 garlic clove, finely chopped
½ teaspoon chopped fresh basil
1 teaspoon chopped fresh parsley
freshly ground black pepper

1 tablespoon cornflour
1 tablespoon water
Crumble
50g (2 oz) plain white flour
4 teaspoons margarine

1   Remove the skin from the fish, and cut the fish into strips about 3.5cm (1½ in) across. Set aside.
2   Place the onion, carrot, beans, tomatoes, garlic, basil and parsley in a saucepan. Add the fish and pepper to taste.
3   Bring the mixture to the boil, cover and reduce the heat. Simmer for 12–15 minutes.
4   Preheat the oven to 180°C/350°F/Gas 4.
5   Blend the cornflour to a paste with the water and stir into the fish mixture. Bring to the boil, then transfer to a deep ovenproof dish.
6   To make the crumble topping, rub the flour and margarine together until the mixture resembles breadcrumbs.
7   Sprinkle the crumbs over the fish mixture and bake for 20–25 minutes.

Fish Moussaka   3L   *Serves 4*

225g (8 oz) cod fillets, cooked, skinned and flaked
450g (1 lb) halibut steaks, cooked, skinned and flaked
2 large aubergines
175ml (6 fl oz) vegetable oil
2 tablespoons sunflower oil
2 small onions, finely chopped
400g (14 oz) canned tomatoes, chopped
a pinch of cayenne pepper

a pinch of dried thyme
freshly ground black pepper
1 tablespoon paprika
100g (4 oz) Cheddar cheese, grated
Sauce
25g (1 oz) polyunsaturated margarine
2 tablespoons plain flour
350ml (12 fl oz) semi-skimmed milk
4 egg yolks
1 tablespoon lemon juice

1 Preheat the oven to 190°C/375°F/Gas 5.

2 Cut the aubergine into slices. In a frying pan heat a tablespoon of the sunflower oil over a moderate heat. Add about one-third of the aubergine slices and fry for 3–4 minutes on each side until they are golden brown.

3 Remove with a spatula and allow to drain on kitchen paper. Fry the remaining slices in the same way. Set aside.

4 Heat the remaining sunflower oil over a moderate heat. Add the onion and cook, stirring occasionally, for 5–7 minutes.

5 Stir in the fish, tomatoes and their juice, cayenne, thyme, pepper and paprika. Cook, stirring frequently, for 3 minutes. Remove the pan from the heat and set aside.

6 Arrange one-third of the aubergine on the bottom of an ovenproof dish. Spoon over it half the fish and tomato mixture. Sprinkle half the cheese over the top.

7 Cover with the remaining fish and tomato sauce mixture. Cover with another third of the aubergine. Sprinkle the remaining cheese over the top. Cover with the remaining aubergine slices. Set aside.

8   To make the sauce, melt the margarine in a medium
    saucepan over a moderate heat. Off the heat, using a
    wooden spoon, stir in the flour to make a smooth paste.
9   Gradually stir in the milk, being careful to avoid lumps.
    Return the pan to the heat and cook, stirring constantly,
    for 2–3 minutes until it is very thick and smooth. Leave to
    cool.
10 When the sauce is cool, beat in the egg yolks, and stir in
    the lemon juice.
11 Pour the sauce over the aubergine slices to cover them
    completely. Place the dish in the centre of the oven and
    bake for 35–40 minutes or until the top is golden brown.
    Serve immediately.

Fish Stew with Peppers   123L   *Serves 4*

900g (2 lb) sole fillets, cut into 2.5cm (1 in) cubes
450g (1 lb) small new potatoes, scrubbed
2 tablespoons sunflower oil
450g (1 lb) canned peeled tomatoes
1 red chilli, seeded and finely chopped
2 green peppers, cored, seeded and sliced
2 medium onions, finely chopped
3 garlic cloves, crushed
50ml (2 fl oz) stock
1 teaspoon dried thyme
1 bay leaf

1   Boil the potatoes until just tender. Drain and keep warm.
2   In an ovenproof dish heat the oil and add the tomatoes
    and their juices, and the chilli. Stirring occasionally, cook

for 15 minutes or until the mixture is thick.

3   Stir in the green peppers, onions, garlic, stock, thyme, bay
     leaf and cubes of fish. Cover the pan, reduce the heat to
     low, and cook for 10 minutes, stirring occasionally.

4   Add the cooked potatoes and turn them over in the fish
     mixture. Cover again and cook for a further 5 minutes,
     until the fish flakes easily when tested with a fork.

5   Discard the bay leaf and serve at once.

Frittata 23L *Serves 6*

125g (4½ oz) small new potatoes
125g (4½ oz) shelled broad beans
50g (2 oz) low-fat soft cream cheese
4 eggs
2 tablespoons chopped thyme
freshly ground black pepper
2 tablespoons olive oil
1 onion, peeled and roughly chopped
225g (8 oz) courgettes, sliced
125g (4½ oz) lightly cooked salmon, flaked
125g (4½ oz) cooked, peeled prawns

1   Cook the potatoes and broad beans separately in boiling
     water until just tender, then drain thoroughly. Set aside.

2   In a bowl, whisk together the cheese, eggs, thyme and
     pepper.

3   Heat the oil in a large shallow ovenproof pan. Add the
     onion, courgettes, potatoes and beans. Cook, stirring, for
     2–3 minutes.

4   Add the salmon and prawns, and pour in the egg mixture.

As the eggs cook, push the mixture to the centre to allow the raw egg to flow towards the edge of the pan.

5 When the frittata is lightly set, place the pan under a hot grill for 2–3 minutes until golden brown. Serve with a green salad.

• *Variation:* Substitute mushrooms for the prawns and salmon for a vegetarian alternative.

Haddock Florentine   123L   *Serves 2*

2× 150g (5 oz) haddock portions
225g (8 oz) fresh or frozen spinach, defrosted and drained
2 tablespoons fresh lemon juice
2 lemon slices to garnish

1 Preheat the oven to 190°C/375°F/Gas 5.
2 Place each haddock portion on a piece of foil large enough to wrap round it.
3 Cover each portion with half the spinach and 1 tablespoon lemon juice, then wrap securely in the foil.
4 Bake in the preheated oven for 20–30 minutes.
5 Remove the foil and serve with a slice of lemon to garnish.

Haddock Kedgeree   23L   *Serves 2*

175g (6 oz) unsmoked haddock, filleted and skinned
75g (3 oz) brown rice
½ green pepper, cored, seeded and chopped
1 small onion, finely chopped
1 tablespoon sunflower oil

1 hard-boiled egg, chopped
1 tablespoon chopped fresh parsley
2 tablespoons low-fat natural yoghurt
freshly ground black pepper
2 lemon slices to garnish

1   Cover the fish with water in a shallow pan. Heat gently and poach for about 8–10 minutes. Remove from the liquid and flake the flesh. Set aside.
2   Boil the rice in the poaching water left in the pan for about 45 minutes (but see cooking instructions on the rice packet). You may need to add extra water.
3   Sauté the green pepper and onion in the oil until softened but not brown.
4   Drain the rice, then stir in the fish, egg, onion, green pepper, parsley and yoghurt and mix well. Heat gently, stirring all the time.
5   Season with pepper and serve garnished with lemon.

Haddock Parcels   123L   *Serves 4*

4 × 150g (5 oz) haddock cutlets
175g (6 oz) courgettes, thinly sliced
225g (8 oz) tomatoes, peeled and thinly sliced
225g (8 oz) celery, sliced
1 red and 1 green pepper, cored, seeded and sliced
100g (4 oz) canned sweetcorn, drained
2 tablespoons lemon juice
2 tablespoons vegetable stock or water
freshly ground black pepper
1 tablespoon chopped fresh parsley

1   Preheat the oven to 180°C/350°F/Gas 4.
2   Place each fish cutlet on a piece of foil large enough to wrap round it.
3   Simmer all the vegetables in the lemon juice and stock for 10 minutes.
4   Separate the vegetables into 4 portions, and pile on top of the fish. Add black pepper and sprinkle with fresh parsley.
5   Wrap the fish up in the foil, and bake in the preheated oven for about 30 minutes.
6   Serve with vegetables or rice.

Halibut Fruit   123L   *Serves 2*

2 halibut steaks, cut in half
finely grated rind and juice of 2 oranges
finely grated rind and juice of 1 lemon
1 orange, peeled, segmented and skinned
orange and lemon slices to garnish

1   Preheat the oven to 180°C/350°F/Gas 4.
2   Place the grated citrus rind in an ovenproof dish with the juices. Add the fish and baste well. This can be left to marinate for 1–6 hours, turning occasionally.
3   Cover the dish with foil and cook in the preheated oven for 10 minutes.
4   Add the orange segments and cook for a further 10 minutes.
5   Serve garnished with slices of lemon and orange.

Hot Fruity Chicken   123L   *Serves 2*

300g (10½ oz) chicken breast, skinned and boned, and cut into strips
1 tablespoon concentrated apple juice
1 garlic clove, chopped
2 teaspoons peeled grated ginger
2 teaspoons chilli sauce
2 teaspoons sunflower oil
150g (5 oz) onions, sliced
1 medium green pepper, cored, seeded and chopped
1 teaspoon cornflour
freshly ground black pepper
2 large oranges, peeled, segmented and skinned

1   Mix together the apple juice, half the garlic, the ginger and the chilli sauce. Add the chicken and coat thoroughly. Cover and refrigerate for at least 1 hour to marinate. It can be left overnight. Remove the chicken and reserve the marinade.

2   Heat the oil in a large frying pan and sauté the onions and remaining garlic until the onion is translucent.

3   Add the chicken and chopped pepper, and cook until the chicken is lightly browned on both sides.

4   Strain the reserved marinade and mix it with the cornflour and black pepper to taste.

5   Add the cornflour mixture to the pan. Bring to the boil, stirring constantly. Reduce the heat to a simmer.

6   Add the orange segments and heat thoroughly, stirring occasionally. Serve immediately.

Japanese Sardines   123L   *Serves 4*

450g (1 lb) fresh sardines, cleaned, washed thoroughly in cold water and dried
115ml (4 fl oz) tamari sauce
50ml (2 fl oz) white wine or sherry vinegar
2 tablespoons lemon juice
25g (1 oz) fresh root ginger, peeled and chopped
2 garlic cloves, crushed

1   In a small mixing bowl, combine the soy sauce, vinegar, lemon juice, ginger and garlic.
2   Arrange the sardines in a shallow baking dish and pour the tamari sauce mixture over them. Leave in a cool place to marinate for 1½–2 hours.
3   Remove the sardines, and discard the marinade.
4   Grill the sardines for 3–5 minutes or longer, depending on the size, turning once. Serve immediately.

Lamb and Apricot Pilaff   123L   *Serves 4*

700g (1½ lb) boned leg of lamb, cut into 2.5cm (1 in) cubes
2 tablespoons sunflower oil
1 medium onion, thinly sliced
75g (3 oz) dried unsulphured apricots, soaked overnight, drained and halved
3 tablespoons organic raisins
½ teaspoon ground cinnamon
freshly ground black pepper

900ml (1½ pints) water
225g (8 oz) long-grain rice, washed, soaked in cold water for 30
  minutes and drained

1 Heat the oil in a frying pan, add the onion and cook for
   about 5 minutes, until translucent but not brown.
2 Add the lamb and cook, stirring and turning occasionally,
   for 5–8 minutes, or until lightly browned all over.
3 Stir in the apricots, raisins, cinnamon, pepper and half of
   the water. Bring to the boil, stirring occasionally. Reduce
   the heat to low, cover the pan and simmer for 1–1¼ hours,
   or until the meat is tender when pierced with the point of a
   sharp knife.
4 Cook the rice in the usual way, using the remaining water.
5 Preheat the oven to 180°C/350°F/Gas 4.
6 Place one-third of the meat mixture in a medium casserole.
   Cover with a layer of one-third of the rice, then top with
   another third of the meat. Continue to make the layers in
   this manner until all the ingredients have been used up,
   finishing with a layer of rice.
7 Cover the casserole and bake for 50 minutes. Serve immediately.

Lamb and Aubergine Bake 123L *Serves 2*

200g (7 oz) minced lamb
1 large aubergine
salt (for the aubergine only)
2 teaspoons vegetable oil
1 small onion, chopped
1 garlic clove, finely chopped

15g (½ oz) cooked brown rice
1 tablespoon canned sweetcorn
1 tablespoon tomato purée
freshly ground black pepper

1   Cut the aubergine in half lengthways. Lightly score inside each half with sharp knife. Sprinkle with salt and leave for 20–30 minutes.
2   Preheat the oven to 190°C/375°F/Gas 5.
3   Rinse the aubergine thoroughly in cold water. Scoop out and chop the white flesh, reserving the hollow halves.
4   Heat the oil in a pan, and gently fry the onion and garlic for 2–3 minutes. Add the white aubergine flesh and stir round for 2 more minutes.
5   Add the rice, sweetcorn, lamb and tomato purée to the pan, season with pepper, and stir for 2–3 minutes to brown the meat.
6   Spoon this mixture into the aubergine halves, cover and bake in the preheated oven for 20–25 minutes. Serve immediately.

Lamb and Parsley Stew   123L   *Serves 4*

450g (1 lb) boned shoulder of lamb, trimmed of excess fat and cubed
2 tablespoons vegetable oil
1 garlic clove, crushed (optional)
1 large onion, sliced
600ml (1 pint) vegetable stock
4 tablespoons finely chopped fresh parsley
1 bay leaf

6 large tomatoes, skinned and chopped
4 tablespoons tomato purée
2 carrots, sliced
1 × 225g (8 oz) can red kidney beans, drained and rinsed
1 tablespoon cornflour, dissolved in 2 tablespoons water

1   Heat the oil in a medium flameproof casserole and then add the garlic, onion and lamb cubes. Fry for 7–8 minutes, stirring occasionally, until the meat is brown on all sides.
2   Stir in the stock, parsley, bay leaf, tomatoes, tomato purée and carrots, and bring to the boil. Cover and simmer for 1 hour.
3   Add the kidney beans and cornflour mixture to the stew and stir well. Simmer for 15 minutes, or until the lamb is tender and the sauce is thick.
4   Remove the bay leaf and serve immediately.

Lamb Kebabs 23L *Serves 4*

450g (1 lb) lamb neck fillet, trimmed and cut into chunks
1 green pepper, cored, seeded and cut into chunks
1 red pepper, cored, seeded and cut into chunks
1 large onion, cut into chunks
450g (1 lb) button mushrooms
lime wedges to garnish
Marinade
3 tablespoons plain yoghurt
juice of ½ lime
2 garlic cloves, crushed
3 tablespoons chopped fresh coriander
1 tablespoon chopped fresh mint

1 teaspoon each curry powder and ground cumin
a pinch of cayenne pepper

1   Combine the marinade ingredients in a large bowl. Add the lamb and stir. Cover and chill for at least 2 hours.
2   Thread the lamb, pepper and onion chunks and mushrooms on to skewers alternately.
3   Cook for 4–6 minutes on each side (either on a barbecue or under a hot grill). Serve with lime wedges.

Lamb in Spicy Yoghurt Sauce   23L   *Serves 4*

900g (2 lb) leg of lamb, boned and cut into 2cm (¾ in) cubes
250ml (8 fl oz) water
1 tablespoon olive oil
3 onions, sliced
freshly ground black pepper
2 garlic cloves, crushed
1 teaspoon chopped fresh parsley
600g (1 lb 5 oz) natural yoghurt
1 tablespoon cornflour mixed to a paste with 2 teaspoons water
1 teaspoon grated lemon rind
1 tablespoon chopped fresh coriander

1   In a large saucepan, bring the water and oil to the boil over a moderate heat.
2   Add the onions, lamb, pepper, garlic and parsley. Cover the pan tightly, reduce the heat to low and simmer for 1¾ hours or until the lamb is very tender and the liquid has reduced by about two-thirds.
3   In a medium saucepan, heat the yoghurt and cornflour

mixture over a moderate heat, stirring constantly. Reduce the heat to very low and cook for 8 minutes or until it has reduced by half.

4   Add the yoghurt mixture and the lemon rind to the lamb mixture, stir well and simmer, uncovered, for 15 minutes.

5   Add the coriander and serve with a salad and boiled rice.

Liver with Orange   123L   *Serves 2*

175g (6 oz) lamb's liver, thinly sliced
1 tablespoon cornflour, seasoned with freshly ground black pepper
1 small onion, thinly sliced
1 tablespoon sunflower oil
½ green pepper, cored, seeded and diced
75g (3 oz) lean bacon, sliced into 2.5cm (1 in) pieces
115ml (4 fl oz) orange juice
2 oranges, segmented and chopped in half

1   Coat the liver in the seasoned flour.

2   Gently fry the onion in the oil in a non-stick frying pan for about 2–5 minutes.

3   Add the pepper, bacon and liver, and fry for a further minute.

4   Add the orange juice and simmer for 5 minutes.

5   Add the halved orange segments, heat through for 1 minute, and serve.

Mackerel with Lemon Stuffing   123L   *Serves 4*

4 × 175g (6 oz) mackerel, split and boned
juice of ½ lemon
freshly ground black pepper
3 tablespoons water
4 slices lemon to garnish
Stuffing
2 teaspoons sunflower oil
1 small onion, finely chopped
125g (4½ oz) cooked brown rice
finely grated rind and juice of ½ lemon
1 tablespoon freshly chopped parsley
1 small egg, beaten

1   Preheat the oven to 160°C/325°F/Gas 3.
2   First prepare the stuffing. Heat the oil in the pan, add the onion and cook for 5 minutes or until golden brown. Transfer to a mixing bowl and combine with the remaining stuffing ingredients.
3   Place the mackerel on a flat surface and sprinkle the flesh with lemon juice and black pepper. Spoon the stuffing into the fish and reshape.
4   Place the fish in an ovenproof dish, and add the water. Cover and bake in the preheated oven for 15–20 minutes.
5   Serve immediately, garnished with the lemon slices.

Poached Halibut with Parsley Sauce   123L   *Serves 6*

6 × 175g (6 oz) halibut steaks
1 small leek, chopped
1 carrot, chopped
2 tablespoons freshly chopped parsley
3 tablespoons lemon juice
150ml (5 fl oz) water

1   Place the chopped vegetables and 1 tablespoon of the parsley over the bottom of a large pan. Add the steaks on top with the lemon juice and water.
2   Bring to the boil, cover and simmer for about 10 minutes. Transfer the halibut to a serving dish and keep warm.
3   Bring the liquid and vegetables back to the boil and simmer for a further 5 minutes.
4   Blend the vegetables to a purée and return to the saucepan. Add the remaining tablespoon of parsley and reduce the liquid until it has thickened.
5   Pour this liquid over the halibut steaks and serve.

Prawn and Vegetable Stir-Fry   123L   *Serves 4*

225g (8 oz) peeled prawns
3 tablespoons vegetable oil
100g (4 oz) broccoli, divided into florets
100g (4 oz) carrots, cut into small matchsticks
100g (4 oz) leeks, thinly sliced
50g (2 oz) courgettes, thinly sliced
100g (4 oz) Chinese leaves, roughly chopped

1 apple, cored and diced
1 tablespoon grated peeled ginger
1 large onion, chopped
1 tablespoon lemon juice

1   Heat the oil in a wok or large frying pan, add the broccoli, carrots and leeks, and stir-fry for 3 minutes.
2   Add the prawns, courgettes, Chinese leaves, apple, ginger, onion and lemon juice, and stir-fry for a further 2 minutes.
3   Serve immediately, with rice.

Salmon and Cheese Roll   23L   *Serves 2*

4 × 25g (1 oz) slices smoked salmon
75g (3 oz) cottage cheese
75g (3 oz) curd cheese
1 teaspoon lemon juice
½ apple, shredded
freshly ground black pepper
2 lemon slices to garnish
50g (2 oz) lettuce, chopped

1   Mix the cottage and curd cheese with the lemon juice and shredded apple. Season with black pepper.
2   Lay each smoked salmon slice on a flat surface and spread with the cheese mixture. Roll up like a Swiss roll.
3   Garnish with the lemon slice and serve on a bed of lettuce.

Salmon Steaks with Ginger   123L   *Serves 2*

2 salmon steaks
2 tablespoons lemon juice
1 × 2.5cm (1 in) piece fresh ginger, peeled and finely chopped
freshly ground black pepper

1   Preheat the oven to 180°C/350°F/Gas 4.
2   Place each salmon steak on a large piece of foil. Add 1
    tablespoon of lemon juice and half the chopped ginger to
    each steak. Season with a little black pepper.
3   Wrap the steaks individually in foil to make two parcels
    and bake in the preheated oven for 20 minutes. Serve hot
    with vegetables or cold with a salad.

Spicy Fish   123L   *Serves 4*

450g (1 lb) cod fillet, skinned and cut into 4 equal pieces
3 large tomatoes, skinned and sliced
1 garlic clove, crushed
½ red pepper, cored, seeded and chopped
½ green pepper, cored, seeded and chopped
1 courgette, thinly sliced
1 onion, thinly sliced
2 teaspoons freshly chopped basil
freshly ground black pepper
a pinch of grated fresh ginger
3 tablespoons lemon juice
2 teaspoons freshly chopped parsley
300ml (10 fl oz) vegetable stock or water

1   Preheat the oven to 180°C/350°F/Gas 4.
2   Place half the tomato slices in a casserole dish and cover with the garlic, red and green peppers, courgette, onion and basil.
3   Season with black pepper and ginger and sprinkle with half the parsley.
4   Arrange the cod on top, with the other half of the parsley, and cover with the remaining tomatoes. Pour on the lemon juice and stock.
5   Cover and cook in the preheated oven for about 40 minutes. Serve immediately.

Steak and Mushroom Pie   3L   *Serves 4–6*

700g (1½ lb) lean stewing steak, cut into chunks
1 large onion, chopped
1 tablespoon sunflower oil
25g (1 oz) cornflour
300ml (10 fl oz) home-made beef stock
½ teaspoon Worcestershire sauce
mixed fresh herbs (rosemary, thyme, marjoram)
freshly ground black pepper
250g (9 oz) button mushrooms
Pastry
50g (2 oz) white Cooking Flora
50g (2 oz) sunflower margarine
225g (8 oz) plain flour
about 3 tablespoons cold water
a little milk to glaze

- The meat mixture can be slow cooked all day or the previous day to allow the flavours to blend and tenderise the beef. Allow to cool and remove fat which will solidify on the surface.

1 Make the pastry first. Rub the fats into the flour until the mixture resembles fine breadcrumbs. Gradually add sufficient water until you have a smooth but not sticky dough. Chill in the fridge for 20 minutes.

2 Sauté the onion in the oil until softened. Add the beef and cook until browned.

3 Add the cornflour and cook, stirring for 1 minute, before adding the stock, Worcestershire sauce, herbs and pepper. Bring to the boil, partially cover, and simmer gently for 1½ hours.

4 Add the mushrooms and cook for 30 minutes or until the meat is tender. Taste for seasoning, then leave until completely cool.

5 When ready to bake and serve, preheat the oven to 200°C/400°F/Gas 6. Roll out half the pastry and use to line a large pie dish. Put the meat filling inside, then cover with the remaining pastry. Pierce the pastry to let the air escape or use a pie funnel.

6 Brush the pastry with milk and bake in the preheated oven for 30 minutes until the pastry is crisp and golden.

Stuffed Mackerel 123L *Serves 2*

2 × 150g (5 oz) fresh mackerel, gutted
1 orange
1 apple, peeled and grated
1 tablespoon finely chopped parsley

1 medium onion, finely chopped
2 tablespoons cooked brown rice
1 teaspoon dried rosemary or 4 sprigs fresh rosemary

1   Preheat the oven to 200°C/400°F/Gas 6.
2   Grate the peel of the orange and chop the flesh into small pieces, discarding the pips.
3   Mix the orange peel, apple, parsley, onion and rice together.
4   Divide the mixture into two and use to stuff the mackerel loosely.
5   Place a little rosemary in each fish, then wrap in foil.
6   Bake in the preheated oven for about 40 minutes.

Sussex Casserole   123L   *Serves 4–5*

900g (2 lb) lean braising steak, cut into 2.5cm (1 in) cubes
900g (2 lb) potatoes, peeled and thickly sliced
2 medium onions, finely chopped
6 celery sticks, trimmed and chopped
450g (1 lb) pickling onions
8 green olives, stoned
freshly ground black pepper
1 teaspoon grated nutmeg
4 whole cloves (optional)
1 tablespoon apple juice
600ml (1 pint) vegetable stock
1 tablespoon cornflour dissolved in a little water

1   Preheat the oven to 180°C/350°F/Gas 4.
2   Cover the bottom of an ovenproof casserole with half the potato slices.

3 Arrange half the steak cubes on top and cover with the onions, celery, pickling onions and olives. Sprinkle with black pepper and nutmeg.
4 Add the cloves (optional).
5 Cover with the remaining steak and potato slices.
6 Mix together the apple juice, stock and cornflour mixture, and pour over the meat, vegetables and potato. Cover and cook in the preheated oven for 2½ hours.
7 Remove the lid and increase the heat to 200°C/400°F/Gas 6 for a further 30 minutes, or until the potatoes are tender and golden brown. Remove from the oven and serve at once. Remove cloves (if used).

Tuna and Fennel Pasta Bake   3L   *Serves 4*

1 × 200g (7 oz) can tuna in brine, drained and flaked
250g (9 oz) white pasta shells
1 tablespoon sunflower oil
1 fennel bulb, trimmed and finely sliced
1 onion, finely sliced
600ml (1 pint) semi-skimmed milk
50g (2 oz) cornflour, dissolved in a little water
freshly ground black pepper
3 hard-boiled eggs, coarsely chopped
50g (2 oz) mature Cheddar cheese, grated

1 Preheat the oven to 200°C/400°F/Gas 6.
2 Cook the pasta in boiling water for 8–10 minutes until just tender. Drain thoroughly and set aside.
3 Heat the oil in a large frying pan, add the fennel and

onion, and cook for 3–5 minutes until softened but not browned. Set aside.

4   To make the white sauce, heat the milk until boiling. Take the milk off the boil and gradually whisk in the cornflour paste, stirring continuously. Add pepper to taste.

5   Stir in the pasta, fennel and onion mixture and the tuna and hard-boiled eggs. Stir in half the cheese and season to taste.

6   Put the mixture into a shallow ovenproof dish and sprinkle the remaining cheese over the top. Bake in the preheated oven for 30 minutes or until heated through and golden brown on top.

• *Variation:* For a tuna and sweetcorn pasta bake, substitute 1 × 200g (7 oz) can sweetcorn and 75g (3 oz) frozen peas, thawed, for the fennel bulb.

Turkey and Chickpeas with Rice   123L   *Serves 4*

900g (2 lb) turkey breast, cut into 2.5cm (1 in) cubes
50g (2 oz) margarine
12 pickling onions
100g (4 oz) chickpeas, soaked overnight and drained
250ml (8 fl oz) vegetable stock
freshly ground black pepper
1 teaspoon cumin seeds
a pinch of turmeric
450g (1 lb) long-grain rice, washed, soaked in cold water for 30 minutes and drained.

1   Boil soaked chickpeas for ½ hour, or until tender.

2   Melt the margarine in a large pan over a moderate heat. Add the onions and turkey cubes and cook, stirring and turning, for 5–8 minutes, until the onions are golden.

3   Add the chickpeas, stock and enough water to cover the mixture completely.

4   Add the pepper to taste, cumin and turmeric to the pan and stir well to blend. Cover the pan and cook for 1¼ hours or until the turkey and chickpeas are tender.

5   Raise the heat and bring the liquid to the boil. Stir in the rice. Cover the pan, reduce the heat and simmer for 15–20 minutes or until the rice is tender and the liquid absorbed.

6   Serve immediately.

Turkey Schnitzel   3L   *Serves 4*

4 × 175g (6 oz) turkey breast escalopes
3 tablespoons plain flour
freshly ground black pepper
1 large egg, beaten
50g (2 oz) fresh white breadcrumbs

1   Preheat the oven to 180°C/350°F/Gas 4.

2   Sprinkle the flour on to a plate and season with lots of black pepper. Pour the beaten egg on to another plate, and sprinkle the breadcrumbs on to a third plate.

3   Coat each escalope with the seasoned flour. Dip each floured escalope into the beaten egg, then dip into the breadcrumbs.

4   Cover and leave in the refrigerator for 30 minutes.

5   Bake the escalopes in the preheated oven for 30–40 minutes until they are cooked through and the breadcrumbs are golden brown.

Winter Chicken   123L   *Serves 4*

4 chicken breasts, skin removed
1 tablespoon olive oil
50g (2 oz) lean back bacon, roughly chopped
1 large onion, cut into small wedges
450g (1 lb) carrots, cut into chunks
450g (1 lb) celery, cut into chunks
200ml (7 fl oz) apple juice
1 × 400g (14 oz) can butter beans, drained and rinsed
freshly ground black pepper
1 bunch watercress
1–2 tablespoons lemon juice

1   Preheat the oven to 180°C/350°F/Gas 4.
2   Cut the chicken into bite-sized pieces and sauté in the oil in a frying pan. Add the bacon and cook until the chicken and bacon are lightly browned.
3   Remove the meat from the pan and place into a large ovenproof casserole.
4   Add the vegetables to the pan and sauté for 5 minutes until lightly browned.
5   Mix in the apple juice, butter beans and pepper to taste. Combine with the chicken and bacon, and cook in the preheated oven for about 45 minutes until the chicken and vegetables are cooked through.
6   Remove from the oven, stir in the watercress and lemon juice, and serve with potatoes of your choice.

Vegetarian Options

Aduki Casserole   123L   *Serves 4*

225g (8 oz) aduki beans, cooked in water and drained
1 tablespoon sunflower oil
1 large onion, sliced
2 celery sticks, chopped
100g (4 oz) carrots, chopped
175g (6 oz) Savoy cabbage, chopped
400g (14 oz) can chopped plum tomatoes
1 tablespoon tomato purée
½ teaspoon ground ginger
50g (2 oz) shelled cashew nuts
freshly ground black pepper

1   Heat the oil in a frying pan and gently fry the onion for 2–3 minutes. Add the celery and carrots and cook for a further 3 minutes.
2   Add the cabbage, tomatoes, tomato purée and ginger, and simmer for 10 minutes.
3   Add the cooked beans, cashew nuts and black pepper and simmer for a further 5 minutes before serving.

Aubergine, Tomato and Mozzarella Gratin 23L

Serves 4–6

900g (2 lb) aubergines
salt (for the aubergine only)
1 tablespoon olive oil
1 × 400g (14 oz) can chopped tomatoes
2 teaspoons chopped fresh herbs
1 garlic clove, crushed
225g (8 oz) mozzarella cheese, cubed
a handful of basil leaves
freshly ground black pepper

1   Trim the ends of the aubergines. Cut them lengthways into thin slices. Sprinkle the slices with a little salt and leave to drain in a colander for at least 30 minutes. (This allows the aubergines to 'sweat' out any bitter juices.)

2   Preheat the oven to 200°C/400°F/Gas 6.

3   Rinse the aubergines thoroughly in water and pat dry with kitchen paper. Heat the oil in a non-stick frying pan and fry the aubergine slices in batches for 3–4 minutes each side, or until golden brown and just cooked through. Drain well on kitchen paper.

4   Spread half the tomatoes and their liquid in the base of a large gratin dish, cover with half the aubergine slices and scatter over half the mozzarella. Cover with the remaining aubergine slices and sprinkle with the basil leaves and pepper to taste.

5   Spread the remaining tomato and juice over the aubergines and top with the rest of the mozzarella. Bake in the

preheated oven for 30–35 minutes or until golden brown and bubbling.

6   Serve with a mixed green salad.

Baked Nutty Onions   23L   *Serves 4*

1 large onion, sliced
1 bay leaf
300ml (10 fl oz) semi-skimmed milk
25g (1 oz) sunflower margarine
25g (1 oz) rice or potato flour
freshly ground black pepper
1 teaspoon ground nutmeg
150g (5 oz) unsalted peanuts, finely chopped
2 tomatoes

1   Preheat the oven to 190°C/375°F/Gas 5.
2   Place the onion, bay leaf and milk in a saucepan and bring to the boil. Cover and simmer for 10 minutes.
3   Strain the milk into a jug, discard the bay leaf and place the onion in a greased casserole.
4   Melt the margarine in a small pan. When foaming, stir in the flour and cook for 1 minute. Gradually add the warm milk, stirring continuously. Cook until thick and smooth. Add the pepper and nutmeg to taste.
5   Pour the sauce over the onions and sprinkle evenly with nuts. Bake in the preheated oven for 20–30 minutes. Reduce the heat if the nuts are browning too quickly.
6   Meanwhile halve and grill the tomatoes. Use as a garnish.

Bean and Tomato Hotpot   123L   *Serves 4*

1 × 415g (15 oz) can red kidney beans, drained and rinsed
1 × 400g (14 oz) can tomatoes
2 tablespoons sunflower oil
2 onions, sliced
3 carrots, sliced
2 celery sticks, sliced
1 large leek, sliced
2 garlic cloves, crushed
300ml (10 fl oz) stock
freshly ground black pepper
700g (1½ lb) potatoes, thinly sliced
15g (½ oz) margarine

1   Preheat the oven to 180°C/350°F/Gas 4.
2   Heat the oil in a flameproof casserole, add the onions and fry for 5 minutes. Add the carrots, celery, leek and garlic and fry for a further 5 minutes.
3   Add the kidney beans, tomatoes with their juices, stock and pepper to taste. Mix well.
4   Arrange the potatoes neatly on top, sprinkling pepper between each layer. Dot with margarine, cover and cook in the preheated oven for 2 hours.
5   Remove the lid 30 minutes before the end of cooking to allow the potatoes to brown.

Butter Bean Biryani   123L   *Serves 4*

175g (6 oz) canned butter beans, drained and rinsed
1 tablespoon sunflower oil
1 medium onion, finely chopped
200g (7 oz) long-grain rice, washed and drained
2 teaspoons curry powder (hot, medium or mild to taste)
1 large red pepper, cored, seeded and diced
1 medium aubergine, diced
2 teaspoons caraway seeds
½ teaspoon finely chopped red chilli pepper
4 cardamom pods
1 × 400g (14 oz) can chopped tomatoes
4 tablespoons canned sweetcorn, drained

1   Heat the oil in a large saucepan, and cook the onion for 2–3 minutes. Add the rice and cook for a further 2 minutes.

2   Mix the curry powder with a tablespoon of water and add to the rice. Then add the red pepper, aubergine, caraway seeds, chilli pepper and cardamom pods. Stir well over a low heat for a further 2 minutes.

3   Drain the tomatoes, keep the juice to one side and add the tomatoes to the rice mixture.

4   Make the tomato juice up to 600ml (1 pint) with water and add to the rice mixture. Cover and simmer for 20 minutes.

5   Add the butter beans and sweetcorn, cover and continue to simmer for a further 10–15 minutes, until the rice is cooked. Remove the cardamom pods before serving.

Cheesy Brown Rice Pie   23L   *Serves 6*

175g (6 oz) brown rice, cooked
250g (9 oz) mature Cheddar cheese, grated
4 tablespoons grated Parmesan cheese
2 spring onions, chopped
2 courgettes, grated
1 red pepper, cored, seeded and diced
1 × 300g (10½ oz) can cut asparagus, drained and chopped
3 tablespoons pine kernels, toasted
3 eggs, lightly beaten
200g (7 oz) natural yoghurt
freshly ground black pepper

1   Preheat the oven to 190°C/375°F/Gas 5.
2   Combine all the ingredients in a bowl and mix well. Season to taste with pepper.
3   Turn the mixture into a greased 23cm (9 in) spring-form tin, and bake in the preheated oven for 40 minutes until firm and golden.
4   Leave in the tin for 5 minutes before removing. Serve hot or cold (it's ideal for picnics).

Chestnut Loaf   3L   *Serves 6*

225g (8 oz) frozen chestnuts, thawed
1 tablespoon olive oil
1 onion, coarsely chopped
2 celery sticks, chopped
2 garlic cloves, crushed

225g (8 oz) potatoes, boiled and mashed
100g (4 oz) fresh white breadcrumbs
1 egg, beaten
2 tablespoons chopped fresh parsley
1 tablespoon soy sauce
1 tablespoon tomato purée
freshly ground black pepper

1   Preheat the oven to 180°C/350°F/Gas 4.
2   Coarsely chop half the chestnuts, and finely chop the remainder.
3   Heat the oil in a pan and add the onion, celery and garlic and cook, stirring, for 3–5 minutes until soft.
4   Remove from the heat. Stir in all the chestnuts, potatoes, breadcrumbs, egg, parsley, soy sauce and tomato purée. Season to taste with pepper.
5   Lightly grease a 1kg (2¼ lb) loaf tin, spoon in the mixture, and level the top. Cover with foil and bake in the preheated oven for 1 hour or until firm.
6   Turn out and cut into slices. Serve hot or cold.

Corn Pasta Italiano   23L   *Serves 4*

285g (10 oz) corn pasta
100g (4 oz) soya mince (textured vegetable protein)
200ml (7 fl oz) vegetable stock
50g (2 oz) vegetarian cheese, grated
4 sprigs parsley
Tomato sauce
2 teaspoons olive oil
100g (4 oz) onion, finely chopped

1 garlic clove, crushed
400g (14 oz) fresh ripe tomatoes, chopped and skin removed, or 1
    × 400g (14 oz) can plum tomatoes, drained and chopped
1–2 teaspoons dried mixed herbs or dried basil
freshly ground black pepper

1   For the sauce, heat the oil in a pan, add the onion and
    garlic, cover, and cook gently for 5 minutes until the onion
    is soft. Add the tomatoes and herbs. Cover and cook for 15
    minutes. Season with pepper.
2   Add the soya mince and the vegetable stock to the tomato
    sauce. Simmer for 10 minutes.
3   Cook the pasta in boiling water as directed on the packet.
4   Drain the pasta and divide between 4 dishes. Pour the
    sauce over the pasta, and top with the grated cheese and
    sprigs of parsley.

Falafel with Sesame Yoghurt Dressing   3L   *Serves 4–6*

1 × 400g (14 oz) can chickpeas, drained and rinsed
6 spring onions, finely chopped
25g (1 oz) white breadcrumbs
1 egg, lightly beaten
finely grated zest and juice of 1 lemon
1 garlic clove, crushed
2 tablespoons fresh coriander leaves
2 tablespoons fresh chopped parsley
1 tablespoon tahini (sesame paste)
1 teaspoon ground coriander
1 teaspoon ground cumin
½ teaspoon ground cinnamon

a pinch of cayenne pepper
freshly ground black pepper
sunflower oil for deep-frying
Sesame Yoghurt Dressing
4 tablespoons natural yoghurt
2 tablespoons olive oil
1 tablespoon lemon juice
1 tablespoon tahini
freshly ground black pepper

1   In a food processor, purée the chickpeas and all the other ingredients (except the oil) until smooth.
2   Turn into a bowl, cover, and leave to stand for at least 30 minutes.
3   Meanwhile, make the sesame yoghurt dressing. In a bowl, combine the yoghurt, oil, lemon juice, tahini and pepper to taste. Cover and set aside.
4   Shape the falafel mixture into balls about the size of walnuts, then flatten them into patties.
5   In a deep-fat fryer, heat the oil to 190°C/375°/Gas 5. (Ensure the oil reaches this temperature so that a minimum amount of it is absorbed during cooking.) Lower the falafel into the fryer in batches and cook for 2–3 minutes until golden. Lift out and drain on paper towels.
6   Serve warm with pitta bread, and the sesame yoghurt dressing.

Mediterranean Vegetable and Egg Grill 23L *Serves 4*

1 tablespoon olive oil
350g (12 oz) courgettes, sliced
1 medium green pepper, cored, seeded and roughly chopped
1 onion, peeled and sliced
1 garlic clove, crushed
freshly ground black pepper
2 teaspoons chopped rosemary
1 × 400g (14 oz) can chopped tomatoes
4 eggs
50g (2 oz) Cheddar cheese, grated

1   Heat the oil in a large frying pan. Add the courgettes, pepper and onion and cook until beginning to soften and brown, stirring occasionally.
2   Stir in the garlic, black pepper, rosemary and tomatoes with their juices. Simmer, uncovered, until the vegetables are tender and the liquid is well reduced, about 20 minutes.
3   Make four slight hollows in the vegetable mixture and carefully break an egg into each. Season the eggs with pepper and top with the grated cheese.
4   Cook under a preheated grill for about 10 minutes, depending on how well cooked you like your eggs.

Mexican Omelette   123L   *Makes 2*

6 eggs
2 tablespoons water
2 tablespoons sunflower oil
Filling
1 tablespoon olive oil
1 onion, finely chopped
1 garlic clove, finely crushed
1 green pepper, cored, seeded and finely chopped
2 ripe tomatoes, skinned, seeded and chopped
125g (4½ oz) button mushrooms, thinly sliced
1 × 225g (8 oz) can spicy mixed beans (one without modified starch)
freshly ground black pepper

1   Make the filling first. Heat the oil in a frying pan, add the onion and garlic and cook for 5 minutes or until softened. Add the pepper and cook, stirring, for 5 minutes.
2   Add the tomatoes and mushrooms and cook, stirring, for 10 minutes. Add the can of mixed beans, and pepper to taste, and simmer for 5 minutes. Keep warm.
3   Beat 3 of the eggs with 1 tablespoon of the measured water. Heat half of the oil in the frying pan.
4   When the oil is hot enough add the eggs, cooking over a medium heat, pulling back the edge as the eggs set, tilting the pan to allow the uncooked egg to run to the side of the pan. Continue until slightly set and golden.
5   Spoon half of the filling on to the half of the omelette farthest away from the pan handle. With a palette knife, lift

the uncovered half of the omelette and flip it over the filling.

6   Slide the omelette on to a warmed plate.
7   Make the second omelette in the same way.

Mexican Stuffed Eggs   123L   *Serves 6*

6 eggs, hard-boiled
1 medium avocado, peeled, stoned and chopped
1 small onion, finely minced
1 small green pepper, cored, seeded and finely minced
100g (4 oz) prawns or shrimps, shelled, deveined and finely
    chopped, or 100g (4 oz) almond halves, finely chopped
1 teaspoon lemon juice
1 teaspoon white wine vinegar
freshly ground black pepper
a pinch of cayenne pepper
1 tablespoon chopped fresh parsley

1   Slice the eggs in half lengthways and scoop out the yolks. Set the whites aside. Using the back of a wooden spoon rub the yolks and the avocado flesh through a fine nylon strainer into a medium-sized mixing bowl. Stir in the minced onion, green pepper and chopped prawns or nuts.
2   Add the lemon juice, vinegar, pepper and cayenne, mixing well to blend.
3   With a teaspoon, generously stuff the egg white halves with the mixture. Arrange on a serving dish, sprinkle with parsley and chill well before serving.

Mixed Vegetable and Almond Stir-fry   123L   *Serves 4*

450g (1 lb) fresh broccoli
225g (8 oz) cauliflower
1 tablespoon sunflower oil
2.5cm (1 in) fresh root ginger, sliced and finely shredded
100g (4 oz) flaked almonds
2 large carrots, peeled and sliced
½ teaspoon sesame oil
225g (8 oz) fresh beansprouts
225g (8 oz) Chinese leaves or white cabbage, shredded

1   Separate the broccoli heads into small florets and peel and slice the stems. Separate the cauliflower into florets and slice the stems.
2   Heat the oil in a large wok or frying pan. When it is moderately hot add the ginger shreds. Stir-fry for a few seconds, then add the almonds and stir-fry until they are lightly browned.
3   Add the carrots, cauliflower and broccoli and stir-fry for 2–3 minutes, then add the sesame oil.
4   Add the beansprouts and Chinese leaves, and stir-fry for about 5 minutes.
5   Serve with noodles or rice.

Nut and Vegetable Loaf   123L   *Serves 4–6*

225g (8 oz) mixed nuts (hazels, almonds, Brazils), finely chopped
  or minced
2 teaspoons sunflower oil
1 small onion, chopped
1 small carrot, chopped
1 celery stick, chopped
1 tablespoon tomato purée
225g (8 oz) tomatoes, skinned and chopped
2 eggs
1 tablespoon chopped fresh parsley
freshly ground black pepper
To garnish
onion rings
parsley sprigs

1   Preheat the oven to 220°C/425°F/Gas 7.
2   Melt the oil in a pan, and add the onion, carrot and celery
    and cook until softened. Add the tomato purée and toma-
    toes and cook for 5 minutes.
3   Put the eggs, parsley and pepper in a bowl and beat well.
    Stir in the nuts and vegetables.
4   Transfer to a greased 900ml (1½ pint) ovenproof dish and
    bake in the preheated oven for 30–35 minutes.
5   Turn out and decorate with onion rings and parsley. Serve
    hot with vegetables, or cold with salad.

Nutty Quorn Risotto   123L   *Serves 4*

225g (8 oz) brown rice
1 tablespoon sunflower oil
1 medium onion, finely chopped
1 clove garlic, crushed
1 red pepper, cored, seeded and sliced
1 green pepper, cored, seeded and sliced
50g (2 oz) green beans, trimmed and finely sliced
100g (4 oz) carrots, cut into matchsticks
100g (4 oz) courgettes, thinly sliced
100g (4 oz) broccoli, broken into florets, stalks sliced
225g (8 oz) Quorn pieces
1 small seedless orange, peeled, divided into skinless segments
1 tablespoon flaked almonds
1 tablespoon chopped fresh parsley
freshly ground black pepper

1   Cook the rice as directed on the packet and put to one side.
2   Heat the oil in a large frying pan and add the onion, garlic,
    red and green peppers and gently fry for 2–3 minutes.
3   Steam the beans, carrots, courgettes and broccoli over a pan
    of boiling water for 10 minutes and add them to the frying
    pan. (Alternatively, if you like your vegetables crunchy, add
    them straight into the frying pan without steaming.)
4   Add the Quorn, orange segments, flaked almonds, parsley
    and rice, plus pepper to taste, and mix and heat through
    until all the ingredients are hot. Serve immediately.

Nutty Sprout Stir-fry   123L   *Serves 2–4*

75g (3 oz) unsalted peanuts
1 medium orange, peeled and divided into segments
2 teaspoons sunflower oil
a pinch of cayenne
½ teaspoon ground cumin
2 thick spring onions, trimmed and sliced
1 garlic clove, thinly sliced
175g (6 oz) Brussels sprouts, trimmed and thinly sliced
1 red pepper, cored, seeded and thinly sliced
2 tablespoons wheat-free soy or tamari sauce

1   Preheat the oven to 190°C/375°F/Gas 5.
2   Place the peanuts on a baking dish in the preheated oven until they are lightly roasted, about 15 minutes.
3   Slice the orange segments crossways into triangles. Set aside.
4   Heat the oil in a wok or heavy frying pan. Add the cayenne, cumin, spring onions, garlic and sprouts and toss in the oil for 1 minute.
5   Add the roasted peanuts and the red pepper, mix and fry again for 1 minute.
6   Lastly, add the orange triangles and soy or tamari sauce and stir-fry until the oranges are heated through. Serve immediately, with rice.

Oaty Chestnut Flan   23L   *Serves 8*

This unusual flan case is not only simple to make, but it can be made in advance and frozen.

Pastry
1 × 435g (15½ oz) can chestnut purée
50g (2 oz) polyunsaturated margarine
150g (5 oz) porridge oats
2 teaspoons dried mixed herbs
Filling
225g (8 oz) potato, cut into chunks
225g (8 oz) leeks, cut into chunks
225g (8 oz) parsnips, cut into chunks
1 red pepper, cored, seeded and sliced
1 bouquet garni
50g (2 oz) polyunsaturated margarine
1 garlic clove, crushed
50g (2 oz) cornflour
75g (3 oz) Cheddar cheese, grated
2 small courgettes, thinly sliced
2 tablespoons chopped chives
freshly ground black pepper

1   Preheat the oven to 180°C/350°F/Gas 4.
2   First make the pastry. In a bowl, cream the chestnut purée with the margarine until smooth, then stir in the porridge oats and herbs. Press the mixture into the base and sides of a 25cm (10 in) round flan dish. Place in the preheated oven and cook for 25–30 minutes or until crisp. Set aside.

3 Now make the filling. Bring 600ml (1 pint) water to the boil in a saucepan. Add the potato, leeks, parsnips, red pepper and bouquet garni. Cover and simmer for about 10 minutes or until the vegetables are tender. Drain in a colander, reserve the liquid and make up to 600ml (1 pint) with water if necessary. Discard the bouquet garni.

4 Heat the margarine in a saucepan and fry the garlic for 1 minute. Remove from the heat and stir in the cornflour.

5 Return to the heat and cook for 2 minutes, stirring. Gradually add the reserved liquid, and bring to the boil, stirring all the time. Simmer for 2–3 minutes, stirring.

6 Add the cheese, cooked vegetables, courgettes and chives and season with black pepper.

7 Spoon the vegetable mixture on to the flan case and serve at once.

• *Variation:* Adapt this recipe by substituting vegetables which are in season.

Oaty Vegetable Crumble   23L   *Serves 4*

Crumble
50g (2 oz) polyunsaturated margarine
50g (2 oz) rice flour
50g (2 oz) porridge oats
50g (2 oz) Cheddar cheese, grated
freshly ground black pepper
Filling
50g (2 oz) margarine
1 onion, sliced
225g (8 oz) celery, sliced

225g (8 oz) carrots, sliced
2 tablespoons rice flour
600ml (1 pint) vegetable stock
225g (8 oz) French beans, halved
225g (8 oz) courgettes, sliced
2 tablespoons chopped fresh parsley
1 × 400g (14 oz) can red kidney beans, drained and rinsed

1   Preheat the oven to 190°C/375°F/Gas 5.
2   To make the crumble, rub the margarine into the rice flour until the mixture resembles fine breadcrumbs. Stir in the oats, cheese and black pepper. Set aside while you make the filling.
3   Melt the margarine in a saucepan, add the onion and fry gently for 5 minutes until softened. Add the celery and carrots, cover and cook gently for 5 minutes.
4   Add the rice flour and cook gently, stirring, for 1–2 minutes. Remove from the heat and gradually blend in the stock. Return to the heat, bring to the boil, stirring constantly, then simmer for 5 minutes. Season with freshly ground black pepper.
5   Add the French beans and simmer for 5 minutes, then add the courgettes and parsley. Cook for a further 5 minutes or until the vegetables are just tender. Add the kidney beans and heat through. Turn the mixture into a deep ovenproof dish.
6   Pile the crumble mixture over the vegetables and bake in the preheated oven for 35–40 minutes or until golden brown.

Polenta with Grilled Vegetables   123L   *Serves 4–6*

175g (6 oz) polenta
150ml (5 fl oz) cold water
600ml (1 pint) boiling water
25g (1 oz) butter
2 courgettes, halved and thickly sliced lengthways
1 fennel bulb, trimmed and quartered lengthways
2 tomatoes, cored and sliced
1 aubergine, halved and sliced lengthways
1 red pepper, cored, seeded, and sliced
1 green pepper, cored, seeded, and sliced
a little melted polyunsaturated margarine
Marinade
2 tablespoons olive oil
2 tablespoons red wine vinegar
2 garlic cloves, crushed
2–3 tablespoons chopped parsley
freshly ground black pepper

* **Variation:** You can adapt this recipe by using marinade 2
  below.

1 Put the polenta into a saucepan, cover with the measured
   cold water, and leave to stand for 5 minutes.
2 Add the boiling water to the polenta, return to the boil,
   and simmer for 10–15 minutes, stirring until smooth and
   thickened. Stir the butter into the polenta.
3 Sprinkle a baking tray with water. Spread the polenta over
   the tray in a 1cm (½ in) layer. Leave to cool.
4 To make the marinade, combine the oil, vinegar, garlic,

parsley and pepper, and mix well. Add the courgettes, fennel, tomatoes, aubergine and peppers, and leave to marinate in the refrigerator for 30 minutes.

5   Lift the vegetables out of the marinade and cook on a barbecue (or under a grill) for 2–3 minutes on each side.

6   Cut the polenta into strips, brush with melted margarine and cook on a barbecue (or under a grill) for 1–2 minutes on each side until golden. Serve hot, with the vegetables.

Marinade 2
2 tablespoons sunflower oil
2 tablespoons tamari sauce
1 tablespoon clear honey
2 teaspoons Dijon mustard
freshly ground black pepper

Quorn and Vegetable Pie   3L   *Serves 4–6*

1 tablespoon sunflower oil
1 onion, chopped
2 carrots, sliced
450g (1 lb) courgettes, sliced
2 large tomatoes, peeled, seeded and chopped
100g (4 oz) mushrooms, sliced
350g (12 oz) Quorn pieces
2 tablespoons chopped fresh parsley
1 tablespoon chopped fresh marjoram
freshly ground black pepper
Sauce
300ml (10 fl oz) semi-skimmed milk
25g (1 oz) cornflour mixed to a paste with a little water

1 teaspoon English mustard
a pinch of cayenne pepper
Pastry
50g (2 oz) white Cooking Flora
50g (2 oz) sunflower margarine
225g (8 oz) plain flour
about 3 tablespoons cold water
a little milk for brushing

1   Preheat the oven to 200°C/400°F/Gas 6.
2   To make the pastry, rub the fats into the flour until the mixture resembles fine breadcrumbs. Gradually add sufficient water until you have a smooth but not sticky dough. Chill in the fridge for 20 minutes.
3   Heat the oil in a large frying pan and fry the onion until soft. Add the carrots and cook for a further 5 minutes.
4   Add the courgettes, tomatoes, mushrooms, Quorn, parsley, marjoram and black pepper. Cook over a gentle heat for 10–15 minutes until just softened. Set aside.
5   To make the white sauce, heat the milk until boiling. Take the milk off the heat and gradually whisk in the cornflour paste, stirring continuously. Add the mustard and the cayenne.
6   Combine the vegetable and Quorn mixture with the white sauce and set aside.
7   Roll out the pastry and use half to line the base of a large pie dish. Pour in the vegetable filling and cover with the remaining pastry. Brush with milk and bake in the preheated oven for 30 minutes until the pastry is crisp and golden.

• *Note:* To make this pie during Stage 2, you can use the wheat-free pastry recipe on page 313.

Red Lentil and Coconut Smoothy   123L   *Serves 4*

225g (8 oz) red split lentils
100g (4 oz) carrots, sliced
1 medium onion, finely chopped
1 garlic clove, crushed
1 teaspoon paprika
½ teaspoon ground ginger
1 bay leaf
15g (½ oz) creamed coconut, finely chopped
2 tablespoons lemon juice
freshly ground black pepper

1   Wash the lentils and put into a large saucepan with the carrots, onion, garlic, paprika, ginger, bay leaf and 600ml (1 pint) water. Bring to the boil, remove any scum, cover the pan and simmer for 25–30 minutes until the water has been absorbed.

2   Remove the bay leaf and mash the mixture into a smooth paste with a fork. Add the coconut, lemon juice and black pepper, and mix well.

3   Serve hot with vegetables or rice.

Roasted Vegetable and Pasta Gratin   3L   *Serves 8*

450g (1 lb) aubergines, cut into bite-sized pieces
700g (1½ lb) mixed peppers, cored, seeded and chopped
450g (1 lb) squash, butternut or pumpkin, chopped
4 tablespoons olive oil
225g (8 oz) pasta shapes

Sauce

900ml (1½ pints) semi-skimmed milk
50g (2 oz) cornflour mixed to a paste with a little water
2 tablespoons wholegrain mustard
150g (5 oz) low-fat soft cheese with garlic and herbs
100g (4 oz) mature Cheddar cheese, grated
freshly ground black pepper
450g (1 lb) frozen leaf spinach, thawed

1   Preheat the oven to 220°C/425°F/Gas 7.
2   Put the chopped vegetables into a roasting pan with the oil. Roast in the preheated oven for 45 minutes or until tender and charred. Reduce the oven temperature to 200°C/400°F/Gas 6.
3   Meanwhile, cook the pasta in boiling water until just tender (*al dente*). Drain thoroughly.
4   To make the white sauce, boil the milk and remove from the heat. Gradually whisk in the cornflour paste until the sauce starts to thicken. Add the mustard, soft cheese and 50g (2 oz) of the Cheddar cheese. Stir thoroughly until smooth. Season with black pepper.
5   Mix the pasta, roasted vegetables and spinach with the sauce until the pasta and vegetables are evenly coated. Spoon into a shallow ovenproof dish and sprinkle over the remaining Cheddar cheese.
6   Cook in the preheated oven for about 40 minutes, or until golden brown. Serve with a green salad.

•   *Note:* Corn pasta can be used to make this dish suitable for Stage 2.

Root Veggie Bake   23L   *Serves 4*

450g (1 lb) potatoes, scrubbed and sliced
175g (6 oz) carrots, scrubbed and sliced
175g (6 oz) parsnips, peeled and sliced
1 tablespoon chopped peanuts
1 tablespoon fresh chopped parsley
75g (3 oz) Cheddar cheese, grated
Tomato sauce
2 teaspoons, olive oil
1 small onion, finely chopped
1 garlic clove, crushed
400g (14 oz) fresh ripe tomatoes, peeled and chopped, or 1 ×
*   400g (14 oz) can plum tomatoes, drained and chopped*
2 teaspoons dried mixed herbs or dried basil
freshly ground black pepper

1   Preheat the oven to 180°C/350°F/Gas 4.
2   To make the tomato sauce, heat the oil in a small pan, add
    the onion and garlic, cover, and cook gently for 5 minutes
    until the onion is soft.
3   Add the tomatoes and herbs. Season with freshly ground
    black pepper, cover and cook for 15 minutes.
4   Meanwhile, bring the potatoes, carrots and parsnips to the
    boil in a pan of water, simmer for 10 minutes, then drain.
5   Grease a large ovenproof dish. Pour in the potatoes, carrots
    and parsnips. Sprinkle with the nuts and parsley and cover
    with the tomato sauce.
6   Sprinkle the top with cheese and bake in the preheated
    oven for 15 minutes. Serve immediately.

Spanish Omelette Bake   23L   *Serves 4*

225g (8 oz) potatoes, diced
100g (4 oz) carrots, diced
100g (4 oz) broccoli florets
50g (2 oz) leeks, sliced
4 eggs, well beaten
200ml (7 fl oz) semi-skimmed milk
1 teaspoon fresh snipped chives
1 garlic clove, crushed
freshly ground black pepper
2 large tomatoes, sliced
50g (2 oz) Cheddar cheese, grated

1   Preheat the oven to 180°C/350°F/Gas 4.
2   Place the potatoes and carrots in a large pan of water and bring to the boil. Reduce the heat and simmer for 5 minutes. Then add the broccoli and leeks and simmer for a further 5 minutes until they are just cooked. (The broccoli and leeks can be steamed over the potatoes and carrots using a metal colander and saucepan lid.) Drain.
3   Place the vegetables in a 20cm (8 in) greased ovenproof dish.
4   Mix the beaten egg, milk, chives, garlic and black pepper and pour over the vegetable mixture. Cover with tomato slices and sprinkle over the cheese.
5   Bake in the preheated oven for 35–40 minutes until set and golden brown. Serve immediately.

Spanish Rice   123L   *Serves 3–4*

150g (5 oz) cooked rice
3 tablespoons olive oil
2 onions, thinly sliced
2 garlic cloves, crushed
1 green pepper, cored, seeded and thinly sliced
2 red peppers, cored, seeded and thinly sliced
350g (12 oz) mushrooms, thinly sliced
1 × 400g (14 oz) can chopped tomatoes
40g (1½ oz) stoned green olives (optional)
1 teaspoon dried oregano
½ teaspoon basil
freshly ground black pepper

1   Heat the oil in a large frying pan. Add the onions and garlic and cook for 5–7 minutes, stirring occasionally.
2   Add the green and red peppers and cook for 4 minutes, stirring frequently. Add the mushrooms, tomatoes with their juices, olives (if using), oregano, basil and pepper and cook, stirring occasionally, for 3 minutes.
3   Add the rice to the pan and cook for 3–4 minutes, stirring constantly until the rice is heated through, and serve immediately. (It can also be eaten cold.)

Spiced Lentil Cakes 3L *Serves 4*

225g (8 oz) green lentils
1 garlic clove, crushed
2 carrots, peeled and chopped
1 small onion, chopped
2 teaspoons ground coriander
2 teaspoons ground cumin
finely grated rind and juice of ½ orange
3 tablespoons chopped fresh parsley
50g (2 oz) fresh white breadcrumbs
freshly ground black pepper
2 eggs, beaten
50g (2 oz) dry white breadcrumbs, sieved
vegetable oil for frying
parsley
wedges of lemon

1   In a large pan cook the lentils in boiling water for 30–35 minutes. Drain and refresh under cold water. Drain thoroughly again.

2   Meanwhile, heat 2 tablespoons vegetable oil in a frying pan. Add the garlic, carrots and onion. Cover and cook gently, shaking the pan occasionally, for 15 minutes. Cool.

3   Place the lentils and vegetables in a blender or food processor with the coriander, cumin, orange rind and juice, and blend until smooth. Transfer to a bowl, stir in the parsley and fresh breadcrumbs, and season with black pepper.

4   Divide the mixture into 8 portions and form into flat

cakes, pressing firmly to remove any cracks. Dip the cakes first in the beaten egg and then in the dry breadcrumbs. Chill for 30 minutes.

5   Shallow-fry the lentil cakes in hot oil for 3–4 minutes on each side until golden brown. Garnish with parsley and lemon wedges.

Spinach and Egg Bake   23L   *Serves 2*

350g (12 oz) frozen chopped spinach
2 eggs
8 teaspoons single cream
freshly ground black pepper
25g (1 oz) Cheddar cheese, grated

1   Preheat the oven to 180°C/350°F/Gas 4.
2   Grease two 10cm (4 in) ovenproof dishes.
3   Cook spinach, following instructions on the packet. Drain and press in a sieve to remove as much water as possible.
4   Divide the spinach between the two dishes. Make a deep well in the centre of each and break an egg into each well.
5   Spoon 4 teaspoons of cream over each egg, season well with black pepper, and bake in the preheated oven for 20 minutes.
6   Remove from the oven, sprinkle with cheese and grill for 2–3 minutes. Serve immediately.

Spinach and Gruyère Soufflé   23L   *Serves 4*

450g (1 lb) spinach leaves, cooked, or 225g (8 oz) frozen leaf
  spinach, thawed
50g (2 oz) polyunsaturated margarine
3 tablespoons brown rice flour
200ml (7 fl oz) semi-skimmed milk
freshly ground black pepper
3 eggs, separated, plus 1 egg white
100g (4 oz) Gruyère cheese, grated

1   Preheat the oven to 190°C/375°F/Gas 5.
2   Grease a 1.3 litre (2¼ pint) soufflé dish. Put the spinach in
    a sieve and press to remove all water. Chop finely.
3   Melt the margarine in a saucepan, add the spinach and
    cook for a few minutes to eliminate any remaining mois-
    ture.
4   Add the rice flour and cook gently for 1 minute, stirring.
    Remove the pan from the heat and gradually stir in the
    milk. Season with black pepper and bring to the boil
    slowly. Reduce the heat and cook, stirring, until thickened.
    Cool slightly, then beat in the egg yolks, one at a time, and
    75g (3 oz) of the grated cheese.
5   In a large bowl whisk the egg whites until stiff, then fold
    carefully into the mixture. Spoon into the soufflé dish and
    sprinkle with the remaining cheese.
6   Stand the dish on a baking sheet and bake in the preheated
    oven for about 30 minutes or until well risen and just set.
    Serve immediately.

Stuffed Pepper   123L   *Serves 1*

1 medium green pepper, cored, seeded and halved lengthways
50g (2 oz) cooked brown rice
½ apple, chopped
50g (2 oz) canned sweetcorn, drained
50g (2 oz) carrot, shredded

1   Preheat the oven to 200°C/400°F/Gas 6.
2   Steam the pepper halves for 10 minutes.
3   Mix the other ingredients together and use to stuff the pepper halves.
4   Place in an ovenproof dish, cover and cook for 15 minutes in the preheated oven. Serve hot or cold.

Vegetable Curry   123L   *Serves 2*

175g (6 oz) cooked butter beans
75g (3 oz) cauliflower, broken into florets
75g (3 oz) turnip, cut into 2.5cm (1 in) cubes
75g (3 oz) parsnip, cut into 2.5cm (1 in) cubes
75g (3 oz) courgettes, thickly sliced
1 small onion, chopped
2 teaspoons vegetable oil
1 garlic clove, crushed
¼ teaspoon turmeric
¼ teaspoon ground coriander
¼ teaspoon ground cumin
1 teaspoon finely chopped ginger
½ small chilli, seeded and finely chopped

2 tablespoons tomato purée
900ml (1½ pints) vegetable stock

1 Heat the oil in a saucepan. Add the garlic, spices and chilli, and stir over a moderate heat for 2 minutes.
2 Add all the remaining ingredients, mix well and bring to the boil.
3 Cover and simmer for 15 minutes, then for a further 10 minutes without the lid.
4 Serve with brown rice and salad.

Salads

Bean Salad   123L   *Serves 4 as a side salad*

100g (4 oz) dried haricot beans, soaked overnight
100g (4 oz) dried chickpeas, soaked overnight
1 bay leaf
2 sprigs of thyme
100g (4 oz) fresh podded, broad beans
100g (4 oz) canned red kidney beans
1 clove garlic, crushed (optional)
2 tablespoons cold-pressed olive or vegetable oil
1 medium onion, finely chopped
2 tablespoons finely chopped parsley
½ teaspoon cumin seeds, ground

1 Drain the haricot beans and chickpeas, and cover with water in a saucepan. Boil for 10 minutes, then add the bay leaf and sprigs of thyme, and simmer for 1–1½ hours until

tender. Drain and leave to cool.

2   Cook the broad beans for 2–3 minutes, then drain and cool. Drain and rinse the canned red kidney beans.

3   In a large bowl mix the garlic with the oil. Add all the beans together.

4   Stir in the onion, parsley and cumin, and serve.

Bean and Sweetcorn Salad   123L   *Serves 4 as a side salad*

225g (8 oz) French beans, cooked, cooled and cut into 2.5cm (1 in) lengths
1 × 100g (4 oz) can sweetcorn, drained
2 small spring onions, chopped
sesame seeds to garnish

Boil the beans for 5 minutes, then drain and cool in cold water. Drain thoroughly, and mix with the sweetcorn and onion. Sprinkle with sesame seeds.

Beansprout Salad   123L   *Serves 4 as a side salad*

175g (6 oz) fresh beansprouts
100g (4 oz) red pepper, cored, seeded and sliced
1 × 100g (4 oz) can sweetcorn, drained
2 dessert apples, grated
4 spring onions, chopped
freshly ground black pepper

Mix all the ingredients together and serve with the chosen dressing.

Beetroot and Cabbage Salad   123L   *Serves 4 as a side salad*

175g (6 oz) firm white cabbage, shredded
175g (6 oz) red cabbage, shredded
175g (6 oz) carrots, grated
1 small onion, finely chopped
½ red pepper, cored, seeded and chopped
25g (1 oz) sunflower seeds
175g (6 oz) raw beetroot, grated

Mix all the ingredients, except for the beetroot. Add the beetroot just before serving with a dressing of your choice.

Cauliflower and Carrot Salad   123L   *Serves 2 as a side salad*

100g (4 oz) raw carrot, cut into small sticks
100g (4 oz) raw cauliflower, divided into small florets
100g (4 oz) cucumber, chopped
½ level teaspoon mixed herbs

Combine all the ingredients, and serve with a dressing of your choice.

Coleslaw   23L   *Serves 4 as a side salad*

450g (1 lb) white cabbage, shredded
100g (4 oz) carrots, grated
1 onion, sliced
1 tablespoon reduced-fat mayonnaise
1 tablespoon natural bio yoghurt
1 tablespoon finely chopped fresh parsley

Mix the vegetables together, then mix in the mayonnaise and yoghurt. Garnish with the parsley.

Courgette and Cauliflower Salad   123L   *Serves 4 as a side salad*

75g (3 oz) courgettes, thinly sliced
225g (8 oz) cauliflower, divided into small florets
100g (4 oz) red pepper, cored, seeded and chopped
1 apple, cored and chopped
1 teaspoon freshly chopped herb fennel

Mix the vegetables together, garnish with the fennel, and serve with a dressing of your choice.

Fruity Cabbage Salad   123L   *Serves 4 as a side salad*

450g (1 lb) white cabbage, shredded
100g (4 oz) green pepper, cored, seeded and chopped
5 radishes, sliced
1 red and 1 green apple, chopped

1 medium orange, divided into segments and halved
100g (4 oz) melon, cut into chunks

Combine all of the ingredients, and serve the salad on its own or with a dressing of your choice.

Ginger and Carrot Salad   123L   *Serves 4 as a side salad*

175g (6 oz) carrots, grated
2 medium apples, grated
1 teaspoon ground ginger
1 celery stick, chopped

Mix all the ingredients together, and serve the salad on its own or with a dressing of your choice.

Greek Salad   23L   *Serves 4 as a side salad*

½ cucumber, thickly sliced
1 small onion, sliced
4 large tomatoes, sliced
4 black olives
100g (4 oz) feta cheese, drained and cut into cubes
4 tablespoons olive oil
1 tablespoon lemon juice
2 teaspoons chopped fresh oregano
½ small iceberg lettuce, shredded

1   Cut the cucumber slices into quarters and place in a bowl with the onion, tomatoes, olives and cheese. Mix well.

2 Combine the oil, lemon juice and oregano and blend together thoroughly.
3 Place the lettuce in a glass bowl and spoon the salad ingredients on top. Pour the dressing over.

Green Salad 123L *Serves 1 as a side salad*

50g (2 oz) lettuce
8 thin slices cucumber
75g (3 oz) green pepper, cored, seeded and chopped
50g (2 oz) watercress

Combine all the ingredients and serve with a dressing if wished.

Minty Cabbage Salad 123L *Serves 4 as a side salad*

250g (9 oz) white cabbage, shredded
1 medium carrot, grated
1 medium green pepper, cored, seeded and chopped
1 medium red pepper, cored, seeded and chopped
1 large bunch of fresh mint, chopped

Mix all the ingredients together and serve with the chosen dressing.

Oriental Rice Salad   123L   *Serves 4 as a main course, 6 as a side salad*

175g (6 oz) long-grain white or brown rice
175g (6 oz) basmati rice
1 tablespoon sunflower oil
6 spring onions, finely chopped
1 courgette, thinly sliced lengthways
1 red pepper, cored, seeded and thinly sliced lengthways
1 yellow pepper, cored, seeded and thinly sliced lengthways
50g (2 oz) mangetout
100g (4 oz) fresh beansprouts
2 tablespoons tamari sauce
freshly ground black pepper
1 tablespoon lemon juice

1   Cook the white rices in boiling water for 12–15 minutes until tender. Drain, rinse with boiling water, drain again, and set aside. If using brown rice, cook separately for 35–40 minutes (check timing on packet).

2   Heat the oil in a frying pan and add the spring onions, courgette, peppers, mangetout and beansprouts. Cook until just tender and slightly browned.

3   Add the tamari sauce, black pepper and lemon juice. Add the cooked rice, stir well and continue frying until all the grains are evenly coated.

4   Serve either hot or cold.

Root Salad   123L   *Serves 4 as a side salad*

100g (4 oz) celeriac root, peeled and chopped or grated
175g (6 oz) carrots, peeled and chopped or grated
100g (4 oz) parsnips, peeled and chopped or grated
75g (3 oz) beetroot, peeled and chopped

1   Mix together the celeriac, carrot and parsnip.
2   Just before serving sprinkle the beetroot on top of the salad.

Spinach and Avocado Salad   123L   *Serves 4 as a side salad*

*40 English spinach leaves, de-stalked and sliced into bite-sized
   pieces*
200g (7 oz) avocado, peeled and sliced
12 black olives, stoned and quartered
Dressing
2 teaspoons olive oil
1 tablespoon fresh lemon juice
1 garlic clove, crushed

1   Combine the spinach, avocado and olives in a bowl.
2   Mix together the oil, lemon juice and garlic and pour this
     dressing over the salad.

Spinach Salad   123L   *Serves 4 as a side salad*

225g (8 oz) fresh podded broad beans
100g (4 oz) courgettes, thinly sliced
75g (3 oz) carrots, grated

75g (3 oz) baby turnips, grated
50g (2 oz) spinach leaves, coarsely chopped
freshly ground black pepper

Blanch the fresh broad beans for 2–3 minutes, then cool in cold water. Drain well and mix with all the other ingredients. Serve with the chosen dressing.

Summer Salad   123L   *Serves as a side salad*

100g (4 oz) courgettes, grated
75g (3 oz) carrots, grated
75g (3 oz) baby turnips, grated
50g (2 oz) spinach leaves, lightly torn
225g (8 oz) podded broad beans, blanched for 2–3 minutes

Combine all the ingredients and serve with a dressing of your choice.

Tomato and Celery Salad   123L   *Serves 4 as a side salad*

225g (8 oz) tomatoes, each cut into 8 pieces
100g (4 oz) celery, chopped
100g (4 oz) green pepper, cored, seeded and chopped
100g (4 oz) lettuce, shredded
1 tablespoon freshly chopped parsley

Combine all the ingredients and serve with a dressing of your choice.

Waldorf Salad   23L   *Serves 4 as a side salad*

50g (2 oz) shelled walnuts, chopped
1 head curly endive, chopped
2 dessert apples, chopped
2 celery sticks, chopped
1 tablespoon linseeds
freshly ground black pepper

Mix all the ingredients together, and serve with the chosen dressing.

Watercress, Fennel and Lemon Salad   123L   *Serves 4 as a side salad*

1 large fennel bulb, thinly sliced
1 small bunch watercress, washed and trimmed
1 handful parsley, washed, well dried and finely chopped
freshly ground black pepper
1 tablespoon fresh lemon juice
1 lemon, thinly sliced

1   Mix together the fennel, watercress and parsley.
2   Add the black pepper and lemon juice. Stir well.
3   Cut each lemon slice into segments and add to the salad.

Dressings

Basic Dressing   123L   *Serves 4*

2 tablespoons red or white wine vinegar
1 tablespoon balsamic vinegar
freshly ground black pepper
4 tablespoons olive oil

Mix the vinegars with seasoning to taste, and then whisk in the olive oil, until the dressing is well emulsified.

Oil and Fruit Dressing   123L   *Serves 4*

2 tablespoons olive oil
1 tablespoon sesame oil
1 teaspoon mayonnaise
1 teaspoon mustard
juice of 1 lemon or 1 tablespoon white wine vinegar
1 teaspoon apple juice
freshly ground black pepper

Blend all the ingredients together until smooth.

Orange Dressing   123L   *Serves 4*

150ml (5 fl oz) olive oil
2 tablespoons freshly squeezed orange juice
freshly ground black pepper

2 tablespoons chopped fresh parsley
chopped flesh of 1 orange

Mix all of the ingredients together and serve with salad of your choice.

Orange and Herb Sauce   123L   *Serves 4*

This sauce can be used to complement meat, fish or vegetable dishes, and can be made in larger quantities in advance and frozen.

2 teaspoons sunflower oil
1 small onion, finely chopped
175ml (6 fl oz) fresh orange juice
2 teaspoons chopped tarragon
2 teaspoons chopped parsley
freshly ground black pepper
2 teaspoons cornflour, mixed with 1 tablespoon water
1 orange, peeled, segmented, pith removed and chopped

1 Heat the oil gently in a frying pan and fry the onion for 5–10 minutes until softened.
2 Add the orange juice, herbs and black pepper, bring to the boil and simmer for 2–4 minutes.
3 Stir the cornflour paste into the sauce in the frying pan. Bring slowly to the boil and stir constantly.
4 Add the chopped orange segments, heat for 1–2 minutes and serve.

Spicy Lentil Dressing   123L   *Serves 4*

225g (8 oz) red lentils
600ml (1 pint) water
2 teaspoons sunflower oil
1 onion, finely chopped
1 garlic clove, crushed
½ teaspoon ginger (ground or grated root)
½ teaspoon ground coriander
½ teaspoon ground cumin

1   Place the lentils in a saucepan and cover with the measured water. Bring to the boil and simmer for 20–30 minutes until the water has been absorbed and the lentils are swollen. The lentils should look like a thickish purée.
2   Heat the oil in a frying pan and gently fry the onion, garlic and ginger for 4–6 minutes until lightly brown.
3   Add the spices and cook for a further 1–2 minutes.
4   Add the lentils and cook very gently for 4–5 minutes.
5   Serve hot with rice, or cold with salad.

Tomato Dressing   123L   *Serves 4*

2 teaspoons olive oil
1 small onion, finely chopped
1 garlic clove, crushed
400g (14 oz) fresh ripe tomatoes, skinned and chopped, or 1 ×
   400g (14 oz) can plum tomatoes, drained and chopped
½ teaspoon mixed herbs or basil
freshly ground black pepper

1   Heat the oil in a frying pan and add the onion and garlic.
    Cover and cook gently for 5 minutes until the onion is soft.
2   Add the tomatoes and herbs. Cover and cook for 15 minutes.
3   Season with black pepper and cool.

Yoghurt and Mint Dressing   23L   *Serves 4*

150ml (5 fl oz) natural yoghurt
2 tablespoons lemon juice
freshly ground black pepper
2 tablespoons fresh mint, chopped
2 tablespoons chopped fresh parsley

Mix all the ingredients together. Use straightaway or seal and
set aside until needed. Shake again before use.

Desserts

Almond Cake   L   *Serves 4–6*

100g (4 oz) ground almonds
50g (2 oz) potato flour
100g (4 oz) sunflower margarine
175g (6 oz) unrefined caster sugar
3 eggs, well beaten

1   Preheat the oven to 180°C/350°F/Gas 4. Grease a deep
    18cm (7 in) round cake tin.
2   Mix together the almonds and potato flour, lifting the
    mixture with a spoon to aerate it.

3 Cream the margarine and sugar together until light and fluffy. Gradually beat in the beaten eggs, a little at a time.

4 Fold in the almonds and flour mixture and spoon into the prepared cake tin.

5 Bake in the preheated oven until firm to touch but still moist.

6 Leave to cool for 10 minutes before turning out on to a wire rack.

Almond Macaroons   L   *Makes 18 biscuits*

2 large egg whites
175g (6 oz) ground almonds
75g (3 oz) unrefined caster sugar
18 almond halves

1 Preheat the oven to 180°C/350°F/Gas 4, and line a biscuit or baking tray with greaseproof paper.

2 Put the egg whites into a large bowl with the ground almonds and beat well. Continue beating while adding the caster sugar 1 tablespoon at a time.

3 Roll the mixture into 18 balls and flatten each with the palm of your hand. Lay the flattened biscuits on to the trays and place an almond half in the middle of each biscuit.

4 Bake in the preheated oven for 25 minutes or until golden brown. Leave to cool on a wire rack.

Apple Charlotte   123L   *Serves 4*

1 level teaspoon low-fat spread
450g (1 lb) cooking apples, peeled and cored
4 tablespoons honey
75g (3 oz) white breadcrumbs
4 tablespoons diluted apple juice
¼ teaspoon ground ginger

1   Preheat the oven to 180°C/350°F/Gas 4, and lightly grease 4 individual ovenproof dishes with low-fat spread.
2   Slice the apples and arrange half equally between the dishes.
3   Top with half the honey and sprinkle on half the breadcrumbs.
4   Repeat the layers until the ingredients are used up.
5   Pour over the apple juice and sprinkle on the ginger.
6   Bake in the preheated oven for about 1 hour or until the apples are tender and the topping is crisp.

Apple and Cinnamon Cake   L   *Serves 8*

4 large cooking apples, peeled, cored and sliced
100g (4 oz) sunflower margarine
100g (4 oz) brown rice flour
4 eggs, beaten
100g (4 oz) ground almonds
100g (4 oz) unrefined caster sugar
1 tablespoon ground cinnamon
a few drops of almond essence

For the decoration
16 apple slices (approx)
1 tablespoon unrefined caster sugar
½ tablespoon ground cinnamon

1   Preheat the oven to 150°C/300°F/Gas 2, and grease a 20cm (8 in) round cake tin.
2   Put the apple slices in a bowl, cover with cold water and leave to soak for a few minutes.
3   Place the margarine, flour, eggs, ground almonds, sugar, cinnamon and almond essence in a bowl and beat until light and fluffy.
4   Pour half the mixture into the cake tin.
5   Drain the apples. Save about 16 slices for decoration, and place the remainder in the tin. Sprinkle with a little caster sugar.
6   Spread the rest of the mixture over the apples and smooth off the top ready for decoration.
7   Gently push the remaining apple slices into the top of the cake in a circle and sprinkle the top with sugar and cinnamon.
8   Bake in the preheated oven for at least an hour, until cooked through. Allow to cool slightly, then gently ease the cake out of the tin and on to a plate.
9   Serve hot or cold.

Apple and Passionfruit Delight   123L   *Serves 4*

4 large eating apples (about 800g/1¾ lb), chopped
150ml (5 fl oz) water
3 medium passionfruit, halved
1 tablespoon pure concentrated apple juice
1 teaspoon grated orange rind
3 egg whites

1   Place the apples and water in a saucepan and bring to the boil. Cover, reduce the heat and simmer for 5 minutes or until the apples are tender.
2   Add the passionfruit pulp and seeds, apple juice and orange rind and stir well, then leave to cool.
3   Beat the egg whites in a bowl until soft peaks form. Fold this into the apple mixture, and refrigerate for an hour before serving, in one large bowl or individual bowls.

Apple and Tofu Cheesecake   123L   *Makes 12 slices*

Seed pastry
50g (2 oz) dried figs, chopped
1 tablespoon boiling water
25g (1 oz) sunflower seeds
25g (1 oz) pumpkin seeds
25g (1 oz) sesame seeds, toasted
25g (1 oz) ground hazelnuts
½ teaspoon mixed spice
Filling
450g (1 lb) eating apples, chopped

115ml (4 fl oz) water
200g (7 oz) firm tofu, in chunks
1 egg white, whisked
2 tablespoons freshly squeezed lemon juice
1 teaspoon vanilla essence
1 teaspoon ground cinnamon
25g (1 oz) ground almonds
25g (1 oz) brown rice flakes

1   Preheat the oven to 180°C/350°F/Gas 4.
2   First, make the pastry. Put the figs in a bowl, cover with the
    boiling water and leave to stand for 10 minutes.
3   Purée the figs in a blender or food processor.
4   Grind all the seeds to a powder and combine in a mixing
    bowl with the ground hazelnuts and mixed spice.
5   Bind the seed mixture with the figs to make a dough. Add
    a little chilled water if necessary.
6   Roll out and use to line the base and sides of a 23cm (9 in)
    baking tin. Bake 'blind' in the preheated oven for 10
    minutes.
7   To make the filling, combine the apples with the water and
    purée in a blender or food processor. Add the tofu and
    continue to blend until a thick paste is formed.
8   Fold in the whisked egg white, lemon juice, vanilla essence,
    cinnamon and ground almonds.
9   Pour the mixture into the part-baked pastry case and
    sprinkle with the brown rice flakes.
10 Return to the oven at the same temperature for 30 minutes.
11 Serve chilled.

Apple Custard 123L *Serves 4*

450g (1 lb) eating apples, sliced
150ml (5 fl oz) water
½ teaspoon ground cinnamon
2 eggs

1 Preheat the oven to 180°C/350°F/Gas 4.
2 Place the apples, water and cinnamon in a saucepan and cook gently until the apple softens and most of the water is absorbed.
3 Blend in a blender or food processor and allow to cool for 5–10 minutes. Whisk the eggs and add a little at a time to the apple mixture, still in the blender.
4 Pour the mixture into a 20cm (8 in) baking dish and bake for 25–30 minutes until browned on top and firm. Serve immediately.

Baked Apple 123L *Serves 1*

1 cooking apple, washed and cored
1 dessertspoon concentrated apple juice
75ml (3 fl oz) water
a pinch of ground cinnamon

1 Preheat the oven to 180°C/350°F/Gas 4.
2 Score around the centre of the apple in a circle just breaking the skin and place in an ovenproof dish.
3 Mix the concentrated apple juice with the cinnamon.

4   Pour the water into the dish, and pour the apple juice over the apple.

5   Bake in the preheated oven for approximately 50–60 minutes.

6   Serve with bio yoghurt or *fromage frais*.

Banana Cake   123L   *Makes 16 slices*

75g (3 oz) dried dates
100 ml (4 fl oz) water
225g (8 oz) finely mashed banana
1 egg, beaten
75g (3 oz) white flour (or brown rice flour if on Stage I or II)
25g (1 oz) soya flour
50g (2 oz) ground almonds
1 teaspoon bicarbonate of soda
½ teaspoon vanilla essence
150 ml (5 fl oz) bio yoghurt

1   Preheat the oven to 180°C/350°F/Gas 4 and lightly grease and flour a 20cm (8 in) baking tin.

2   Cook the dates in the water over a low heat until all the water has been absorbed. Blend in a food processor to a smooth paste.

3   Mix the cooled paste with the banana and egg, then fold in the flours, ground almonds and bicarbonate of soda. Stir in the vanilla essence and yoghurt.

4   Pour into the prepared tin and bake in the preheated oven for 35–40 minutes or until the cake is brown on top and comes away from the tin.

Banana and Tofu Cream   123L   *Serves 4*

200g (7 oz) firm tofu, chopped
200g (7 oz) bananas, peeled and sliced
75g (3 oz) ground almonds
a pinch of ground cinnamon
2 teaspoons almond flakes

1   Blend or process the tofu and bananas together. To obtain a creamy texture, the mixture may need to be put through a sieve or food mill.
2   Add the ground almonds and mix well.
3   Spoon into four bowls or glasses and sprinkle lightly with the cinnamon and a few almond flakes.

Bara Brith   L   *Serves 8*

This is a dense Welsh teabread, traditionally thickly sliced and served with low-fat spread.

350g (12 oz) mixed dried fruit
150g (5 oz) light muscovado sugar
grated rind and juice of ½ lemon
300ml (10 fl oz) strong hot Redbush tea
150g (5 oz) rice flour
150g (5 oz) potato flour
1 teaspoon wheat-free baking powder
1 egg, beaten

1   Combine the dried fruit, sugar, lemon rind and juice and
    hot tea in a large bowl. Stir the mixture, then cover and
    leave to steep for at least 8 hours.

2   Preheat the oven to 150°C/300°F/Gas 2, and grease a 1kg
    (2 lb) loaf tin.

3   Add the flours, baking powder and egg to the fruit mixture,
    and stir thoroughly until all the ingredients are combined.

4   Pour the whole mixture into the prepared tin and bake in
    the preheated oven for 1½–1¾ hours until slightly risen
    and firm to touch. To check whether it's done, insert a
    skewer into the middle. If it comes out clean, the teabread
    is cooked. If not, return to the oven for a further 10
    minutes.

5   Leave to cool in the tin for 10 minutes, then turn out on to
    a wire rack.

6. Serve sliced with low-fat spread.

Blackberries with Hazelnut Cheese   23L   *Serves 6*

700g (1½ lb) blackberries (fresh or frozen)
1 tablespoon dark soft brown sugar
½ tablespoon tropical fruit juice
50g (2 oz) shelled hazelnuts
1 teaspoon unrefined caster sugar
175g (6 oz) cottage cheese

1   Mix the cleaned blackberries with the brown sugar and
    tropical fruit juice.

2   Toast the hazelnuts in a frying pan and add the caster sugar
    when the nuts are brown. Shake the pan continuously to

coat the nuts in the melting sugar. Set aside on a plate to cool.

3   Grind the caramel-coated nuts roughly in a processor or mortar, and spread them out on a large sheet of greaseproof paper.

4   Divide the cottage cheese into 6 × 25g (1 oz) balls, then roll them in the crushed nuts, gently pressing the nuts on to the surface of the cheese.

5   Place the individual cheese balls on a plate and put into the refrigerator to set.

6   When you are about to serve, place the individual cheese balls in dessert glasses and surround each one with the berries.

Carrot and Date Cake   L   *Makes about 16 slices*

¼ teaspoon sunflower oil
50g (2 oz) polyunsaturated margarine
6 tablespoons honey
100g (4 oz) carrots, peeled and finely grated
100g (4 oz) dates, stoned and chopped
225g (8 oz) brown rice flour
75g (3 oz) ground almonds
1 level teaspoon bicarbonate of soda
½ level teaspoon cream of tartar
½ level teaspoon ground cinnamon
1 egg
115ml (4 fl oz) skimmed milk
3 tablespoons unsweetened orange juice

1   Preheat the oven to 180°C/350°F/Gas 4, and line a 15cm

(6 in) square tin with greaseproof paper. Brush with a little oil.

2 Place the margarine and honey in a small pan and warm until melted.

3 In a bowl, mix together the carrots, dates, flour, ground almonds, bicarbonate of soda, cream of tartar and cinnamon.

4 Beat the egg with the milk and orange juice until blended, then add to the honey and margarine mixture. Pour into the carrot and date mixture.

5 Stir all the ingredients together gently until thoroughly mixed, then pour into the prepared tin. Bake in the preheated oven for 1 hour. Cool on a wire rack.

Christmas Pudding L *Serves 12*

a little oil
100g (4 oz) Flora Cooking margarine
2 eggs, beaten
100g (4 oz) alternative breadcrumbs (wheat, oats, rye and barley free)
50g (2 oz) brown rice flour
50g (2 oz) cornflour
100g (4 oz) molasses
1 large cooking apple, chopped
1 teaspoon ground cinnamon
1 teaspoon ground ginger
1 teaspoon mixed spice
225g (8 oz) organic raisins
100g (4 oz) organic sultanas

100g (4 oz) organic currants
50g (2 oz) mixed candied peel
1 carrot, grated
50g (2 oz) flaked almonds
zest of 1 large orange
zest of 1 large lemon
3 tablespoons rum
3 tablespoons brandy
3 tablespoons port
1 teaspoon wheat-free baking powder
½ teaspoon bicarbonate of soda

1   Lightly grease a 1.2 litre (2 pint) pudding basin with a little oil.

2   In a small pan melt the margarine. Cool, then pour into a bowl.

3   Add all the ingredients, mix together well, and place in the pudding basin.

4   Cover with greaseproof paper and a layer of muslin or cotton. Tie with string, bring the sides of the muslin up and knot to make a handle which will make it easier to lift out of the pressure cooker or pan when cooked.

5   Pressure-cook for 2 hours or steam for 9 hours in a large saucepan half filled with water.

Coconut pyramids   L   *Makes 24*

4 egg yolks or 2 whole eggs
75g (3 oz) unrefined caster sugar
juice and rind of ½ lemon
225g (8 oz) desiccated coconut

1   Preheat the oven to 190°C/375°F/Gas 5, and grease a baking tray.
2   Beat the eggs and sugar together until creamy.
3   Stir in the lemon juice and rind and the coconut.
4   Form into pyramid shapes either with your hands or using a moist egg cup and place on a greased baking tray.
5   Bake in the preheated oven for 20–25 minutes until the tips are golden brown. Cool on a wire rack.

Country Apple Pud   23L   *Serves 4–6*

3 large cooking apples, peeled, cored and sliced
2 tablespoons unrefined white sugar
1 tablespoon water
25g (1 oz) margarine
50g (2 oz) rolled oats
25g (1 oz) brown sugar
1 tablespoon lemon juice
1 teaspoon ground cinnamon
50g (2 oz) organic sultanas
25g (1 oz) organic currants
25g (1 oz) organic raisins
25g (1 oz) chopped nuts

1. Preheat the oven to 190°C/375°F/Gas 5, and grease an 18cm (7 in) square baking tin.
2. Place the apples in a saucepan with the unrefined white sugar and the water. Cook for 5–10 minutes until just soft. Drain.
3. In a pan melt the margarine. Remove from the heat and add the oats, brown sugar and lemon juice. Add the apples and the remaining ingredients. Mix well.
4. Spoon the mixture into the prepared tin and bake for 20 minutes in the preheated oven until golden and firm to touch. Serve with home-made custard.

Cranberry Sorbet   123L   *Serves 4*

225g (8 oz) fresh cranberries
300ml (10 fl oz) unsweetened orange juice
300ml (10 fl oz) water
artificial sweetener to taste if necessary
2 egg whites

1. Place the cranberries, orange juice and water in a saucepan. Bring to the boil, cover and simmer gently for 2–3 minutes.
2. Blend the soft cranberries in a liquidiser with the juices. Allow to cool and add the sweetener, if necessary.
3. Put the cranberry mixture into a shallow dish and place in the freezer until semi-frozen.
4. Whisk the egg whites until stiff.
5. Remove the cranberry mixture from the freezer and break up the ice crystals that have formed. Tip the semi-frozen sorbet into a bowl and fold in the whisked egg white.

Return the mixture to the container and freeze until firm.

6   When you are ready to serve, scoop the cranberry sorbet into dessert glasses.

Dried Fruit Compote   123L   *Serves 2*

100g (4 oz) mixture of organic dried fruits (e.g. peaches, prunes, apples, apricots and pears), washed
5 level tablespoons orange juice
2 whole cloves
2 × 2.5cm (1 in) cinnamon sticks
juice and zest of ½ lemon

1   Place the fruit in a bowl with the orange juice, spices, lemon juice and zest and leave to soak overnight.

2   Next day, if the juice has been absorbed add 2 tablespoons of water. Then place the mixture in a saucepan, bring to the boil, cover and simmer on a very low heat for 10–15 minutes.

3   Transfer to a serving bowl and remove the cinnamon and cloves. Leave to cool or serve warm with bio yoghurt or *fromage frais*.

Flapjacks   L   *Makes 8*

285g (10 oz) polyunsaturated margarine or butter
175g (6 oz) raw brown sugar
75g (3 oz) golden syrup or brown rice syrup
450g (1 lb) porridge oats

1. Preheat the oven to 190°C/375°F/Gas 5.
2. Melt the butter, sugar and syrup in a pan. Do not allow to boil.
3. Remove from the heat and mix in the oats. Stir well.
4. Press into a shallow square tin, and smooth the surface. Bake in the preheated oven for 25–30 minutes.
5. Mark into portions while still warm, then cool on a wire tray. Cut into individual flapjacks when cold.

Fresh Fruit Salad 123L *Serves 4*

1 dessert apple, peeled and sliced
1 banana, peeled and sliced
4 tablespoons lemon juice
1 orange, peeled and segmented
1 grapefruit, peeled and segmented
100g (4 oz) seedless grapes
2 kiwi fruit, peeled and sliced
2 tablespoons orange juice
4 sprigs fresh mint

1. Toss the apple and banana in the lemon juice. This will prevent discoloration.
2. Combine all the fruit and juices and chill in the fridge.
3. Serve in individual dishes, each one decorated with a sprig of mint.

Fruit Snow 123L *Serves 2*

200g (7 oz) dessert apples, peeled, cored and thinly sliced
2 tablespoons water

grated rind of ½ orange
1 large egg white, beaten until stiff
2 orange slices for garnish

1   Place the apples, water and orange rind in a saucepan. Cover and cook gently, stirring occasionally, until the apple is soft.
2   Rub the apple through a sieve and allow to cool.
3   Fold in the egg white and chill in the fridge.
4   Serve in individual dishes, each garnished with a slice of orange.

Ginger Cake L *Serves 8–10*

100g (4 oz) sunflower margarine
75g (3 oz) dark muscovado sugar
150ml (5 fl oz) golden syrup or brown rice syrup
150ml (5 fl oz) molasses
2 teaspoons ground ginger
½ teaspoon mixed spice
50g (2 oz) maize meal (available from health food shops)
100g (4 oz) potato flour
100g (4 oz) rice flour
½ teaspoon wheat-free baking powder
2 eggs
150ml (5 fl oz) milk

1   Preheat the oven to 160°C/325°F/Gas 3, and grease a 20cm (8 in) round cake tin.
2   In a pan, melt the margarine, sugar, syrup and molasses. Stir in the spices.

3   Sift the three flours together with the baking powder into a bowl and make a well in the centre.
4   Add the syrup mixture to the well and beat until smooth.
5   Lightly beat the eggs and milk together, then gradually beat into the batter.
6   Pour into the prepared cake tin and bake in the preheated oven for 1 hour. (Lemon glacé icing can be drizzled over the top if wanted.)

Gooseberry Jelly   123L   *Serves 6*

450g (1 lb) gooseberries, topped and tailed
150ml (5 fl oz) water
300ml (10 fl oz) pure apple juice
4 teaspoons powdered gelatine (or Gelzone)
2 tablespoons water
Gooseberries to decorate

1   Very sparingly, oil a 900ml (1½ pint) jelly mould.
2   Simmer the gooseberries in the water until soft. Blend in the liquidiser.
3   Mix the purée with the apple juice.
4   Mix the gelatine or Gelzone with the water in a small heatproof bowl, place the bowl in hot water and stir until dissolved.
5   Add the gooseberry mixture to the gelatine mixture and mix thoroughly. Pour into the prepared jelly mould and chill for 2–3 hours until set.
6   Turn the jelly carefully out on to a serving plate and decorate with gooseberries.

Grapefruit Sorbet   23L   *Serves 4*

2 grapefruit
425ml (15 fl oz) water
about 3 tablespoons concentrated apple juice
3 tablespoons natural yoghurt
2 egg whites
peeled grapefruit segments for decoration

1   Thinly pare the rind from the grapefruit. Place the grape-
    fruit rind and the water into a pan. Simmer gently for 8
    minutes and strain into a bowl.
2   Cut the grapefruit in half and squeeze out the juice. Add
    the juice to the liquid from the grapefruit rind and add
    apple juice to taste.
3   Pour the liquid into a shallow freezer container and freeze
    until semi-frozen.
4   Turn the semi-frozen mixture into a bowl and beat to break
    up the ice crystals. Mix in the yoghurt.
5   Whisk the egg whites until stiff and fold gently into the
    grapefruit and yoghurt mixture. Return to the freezer until
    firm.
6   When ready to serve, scoop the sorbet out into dessert
    glasses and decorate with peeled grapefruit segments.

Honey and Sesame Seed Squares L *Makes 8*

50g (2 oz) sesame seeds
100g (4 oz) jumbo oats
75g (3 oz) honey
4 tablespoons sunflower oil
50g (2 oz) sultanas or raisins
25g (1 oz) raw brown sugar

1 Preheat the oven to 180°C/350°F/Gas 4, and grease a 20cm (8 in) shallow square tin.
2 Mix all the ingredients together well and press into the prepared tin.
3 Bake in the preheated oven for 30–35 minutes until golden brown.
4 Cool in the tin then cut into squares and transfer to a cooling rack.

Jellied Grapefruit 123L *Serves 4*

2 large pink grapefruit, halved
300ml (10 fl oz) unsweetened pineapple juice
150ml (5 fl oz) unsweetened grapefruit juice
3 teaspoons powdered gelatine (or Gelzone)

1 Scoop out the grapefruit segments from each grapefruit half. Remove any pith from the segments and from the grapefruit shells.
2 Place the four grapefruit shells on a dish and divide the grapefruit segments evenly among them.

3　Mix together the fruit juices.
4　Take 2 tablespoons of mixed juices and add to the gelatine in a bowl. Place the bowl in hot water, and stir until the gelatine has dissolved.
5　Mix the gelatine liquid with the remaining mixed fruit juice. Pour equal amounts into each grapefruit shell, and place in the fridge to set.

Lemon and Almond Cake   L   *Serves 8–10*

175g (6 oz) sunflower margarine
150g (5 oz) unrefined caster sugar
3 eggs
175g (6 oz) self-raising flour or brown rice flour
50g (2 oz) ground almonds
grated rind and juice of 1 lemon
½ teaspoon almond essence
To finish
2 lemons
2 tablespoons clear honey

1　Preheat the oven to 160°C/325°F/Gas 3. Grease and line a 20cm (8 in) loose-bottomed round cake tin.
2　Place all the cake ingredients in a large bowl and mix well. Beat with a wooden spoon or electric whisk for 2–3 minutes until light and fluffy.
3　Turn the mixture into the prepared cake tin and smooth the top. Pare off the rind and pith of the 2 lemons, then slice the lemons into thin slices and place them on top of the cake.
4　Bake in the preheated oven for 50–60 minutes until golden

and firm. Cool in tin for 10 minutes, then release the sides
and cool on a wire rack.

5   Warm the honey, brush over the cake and serve.

Lemon Fruit Roll   23L   *Makes approximately 10 slices*

½ teaspoon sunflower oil
3 eggs
grated rind of 1 lemon
1 tablespoon concentrated apple juice
50g (2 oz) white self-raising flour
2 tablespoons hot water
4 tablespoons lemon curd
4 rings canned pineapple in natural juice, chopped

1   Preheat the oven to 200°C/400°F/Gas 6. Line a 20 × 28cm
    (8 × 11 in) swiss roll tin with greaseproof paper and brush
    lightly with the oil.
2   Separate the eggs and whisk the yolks with the grated lemon
    rind and concentrated apple juice until light and creamy.
3   Sieve the flour and fold into the egg mixture with the water.
4   Whisk the egg white until stiff and then fold gently into
    the mixture.
5   Pour the mixture into the prepared swiss roll tin and bake
    in the preheated oven for 12–15 minutes.
6   Turn out onto a sheet of greaseproof paper and trim the
    edges.
7   Roll up with the paper inside and leave to cool.
8   When cool, unroll the swiss roll gently and spread with the
    lemon curd and chopped pineapple pieces.
9   Roll up again and place on a serving dish.

Melon Ice-cream   23L   *Serves 4*

1 medium melon (ogen or similar)
300ml (10 fl oz) plain yoghurt
concentrated apple juice to sweeten if necessary
raspberries to decorate

1   Halve the melon, discard the seeds and then scoop out the melon flesh and place in the liquidiser.
2   Liquidise the melon flesh and mix with the yoghurt and concentrated apple juice to taste.
3   Place the melon and yoghurt mixture in a shallow dish and freeze until firm.
4   When ready to serve, scoop the melon ice-cream into dessert glasses and decorate with raspberries.

Millet and Peanut Cookies   L   *Makes 10*

4 tablespoons sunflower oil
1 egg
75g (3 oz) raw brown sugar
100g (4 oz) ground peanuts
75g (3 oz) raisins
100g (4 oz) millet flakes

1   Preheat the oven to 180°C/350°F/Gas 4, and lightly grease a baking sheet.
2   Lightly whisk together the oil, egg and sugar. Stir in the remaining ingredients until well blended.
3   Roll the mixture into 10 balls, place on the greased baking

sheet, and press each one down to flatten slightly.

4   Bake in the preheated oven for about 15 minutes, until golden.

5   Allow to cool on the baking sheet for a few minutes before putting on a cooling rack.

Orange Jelly   123L   *Serves 8*

4 large oranges
2 teaspoons agar powder (or the equivalent of powdered gelatine or Gelzone)
115ml (4 fl oz) apple juice

1   Cut the oranges in half and scoop out the flesh. Put the empty orange halves to one side.

2   Remove the pith and pips from the orange segments and blend the flesh in a blender or food processor.

3   In a small bowl, make a paste by mixing the agar powder with a little of the apple juice. Pour this into a saucepan with the rest of the apple juice, and 2 tablespoons of the blended orange.

4   Bring to the boil and cook gently for 1½ minutes.

5   Take the pan off the heat and add the mixture to the rest of the blended oranges. Mix well.

6   Leave the mixture to cool slightly, then pour it into the 8 orange halves. Leave to set in the fridge.

Pancakes 123L *Serves 4*

1 small egg, beaten
300ml (½ pint) skimmed milk
100g (4 oz) plain white flour

1   Mix together the egg and milk, then sift in the flour, whisking regularly, to make a thin batter.
2   Use kitchen paper to wipe a small non-stick frying pan with a little oil and heat the oil until it is smoking.
3   Pour a generous 2 tablespoons of batter into the pan and swirl it around to cover the base. Cook for a few seconds. Flip it over and cook for a further few seconds. Serve at once.

Passionfruit Fool 23L *Serves 4*

6 ripe passionfruit
150ml (5 fl oz) skimmed milk
3 teaspoons cornflour
2 tablespoons water
150ml (5 fl oz) natural yoghurt
1 tablespoon clear honey

1   Halve the passionfruit and scoop the fruit pulp into a bowl.
2   Gently heat the skimmed milk.
3   Blend the cornflour and water into a smooth paste and then stir into the hot milk. Stir over the heat until the sauce has thickened, then remove to cool slightly.
4   Stir the yoghurt and honey into the sauce and leave until cool.

5   Combine the sauce and the passionfruit pulp and then spoon the mixture into serving dishes.
6   Chill for 3–4 minutes before serving.

Peach Sundae   123L   *Serves 2*

2 peaches
150g (5 oz) raspberries
1 teaspoon arrowroot
2½ teaspoons unrefined caster sugar
2 teaspoons, shredded fresh or toasted desiccated coconut

1   Skin the peaches by blanching them. (Pour boiling water over them, leave to cool briefly, and then place in cold water. The skin will peel off easily.) Halve the peaches and remove the stones.
2   Sieve the raspberries to make a purée. Then take a little of the raspberry purée and mix with the arrowroot into a paste.
3   Stir the arrowroot paste into the remaining raspberry purée, and add the sugar.
4   Place the mixture in a saucepan, bring to the boil and cook for 1 minute, stirring constantly. Remove from the heat and allow to cool.
5   When the mixture has cooled, pour it over the peaches and sprinkle with the coconut.

Pineapple Cake   123L   *Makes 12 slices*

50g (2 oz) prunes, stoned and finely chopped
25g (1 oz) dried figs, chopped

150 ml (5 fl oz) water
285g (10 oz) fresh pineapple or tinned pineapple in fruit juice,
    drained
25g (1 oz) raisins
40g (1½ oz) pumpkin seeds
2 eggs, beaten
40g (1½ oz) ground almonds
75g (3 oz) brown rice flour

1   Preheat the oven to 180°C/350°F/Gas 4, and grease and
    flour a 20cm (8 in) baking tin.
2   Place the prunes, figs and water in a saucepan, bring to the
    boil and simmer until the water has been absorbed and the
    fruit is soft. Put into a bowl, mash with a fork and leave to
    cool.
3   Chop the pineapple into 1cm (½ in) squares, combine with
    the raisins, and add the dried fruit paste.
4   Grind the pumpkin seeds.
5   Add the egg to the fruit mixture, then fold in the ground
    almonds, pumpkin seeds and flour.
6   Pour the mixture into the prepared 20cm (8 in) baking tin
    and bake in the preheated oven for 40 minutes. Cool on a
    wire rack.

Rhubarb and Ginger Mousse   123L   *Serves 4*

450g (1 lb) rhubarb, trimmed and chopped into 25cm (1 in) pieces
3 tablespoons clear honey
juice and grated rind of ½ orange
¼ teaspoon ground ginger
2 teaspoons powdered gelatine (or Gelzone)

2 tablespoons water
2 egg whites

1   Put the rhubarb into a pan with the honey, orange juice and rind and the ginger, bring to the boil and simmer gently until the fruit is soft.
2   In a bowl dissolve the gelatine or Gelzone in the water. Place the bowl in hot water and stir until the gelatine is dissolved.
3   Add the gelatine mixture to the fruit, beat until smooth, then allow to cool until it is half-set.
4   Whisk the egg whites until stiff and fold them lightly into the half-set mixture.
5   Spoon into decorative glasses and chill until set.

Tropical Crumble   23L   *Serves 4*

This topping works very well with any type of fresh fruit.

4 bananas, peeled and sliced
2 tablespoons unrefined brown sugar
2 tablespoons pure maple syrup
50g (2 oz) rice flour
50g (2 oz) porridge oats
25g (1 oz) soft brown sugar
15g (1½ oz) desiccated coconut
50g (2 oz) butter, melted

1   Place the sliced bananas, sugar and maple syrup in an ovenproof dish and cook under a low grill for 3 minutes.
2   Mix the dry ingredients together and pour the melted butter over the mixture. Mix well.

3   Sprinkle the oaty topping over the bananas and grill under
    a moderate heat for a further 3 minutes, until golden
    brown and crunchy.
4   Serve with custard or bio yoghurt.

Walnut Bars   L   *Makes 8 bars*

3 tablespoons sunflower oil
1 tablespoon black treacle
100g (4 oz) raw brown sugar
100g (4 oz) shelled walnuts, chopped
2 eggs
2 teaspoons vanilla essence
100g (4 oz) oats
50g (2 oz) skimmed milk powder
½ teaspoon wheat-free baking powder

1   Preheat the oven to 180°C/350°F/Gas 4, and grease a
    20cm (8 in) square shallow cake tin.
2   Beat together the first 7 ingredients, then sift in the milk
    powder and baking powder and beat well.
3   Pour the mixture into the prepared cake tin and bake in the
    preheated oven for 25–30 minutes until just firm.
4   Cut into bars while still warm.

Wheat-free Pastry   123L
Makes enough to line a 30cm (12 in) flan dish

50g (2 oz) rice flour
50g (2 oz) cornflour

1 egg
50g (2 oz) white Cooking Flora

1   Combine all the ingredients and form into a small ball.
2   Roll out on to greaseproof paper.
3   To keep the pastry intact, place a flan dish face down on to the pastry on the greaseproof paper, and invert.
4   Lightly press the pastry down and around the sides of the flan dish. Fill and bake as directed, depending on which recipe is used for the filling.

Yoghurt Ice-cream   23L   *Serves 4*

225g (8 oz) raspberries, plums, peaches or other soft fruit
1 teaspoon concentrated apple juice to sweeten
285g (10 oz) natural yoghurt
4 mint sprigs to decorate

1   Wash and prepare the fruit as necessary, and purée it in the liquidiser with the apple juice.
2   Spoon the mixture into a freezer container, and put in the freezer for 2–3 hours until semi-frozen.
3   Remove the mixture from the freezer, turn into a bowl and beat to break up the ice crystals. Add the yoghurt and whisk well, then return to the freezer and freeze until firm.
4   Transfer the yoghurt ice-cream from the freezer to the refrigerator 30 minutes before serving to allow it to soften.
5   Scoop the ice-cream into 4 chilled dessert dishes and decorate each one with a sprig of mint.

Bread Alternatives

Cheesejacks L *Makes 8*

150g (5 oz) porridge oats
175g (6 oz) strong Cheddar cheese, grated
1 egg, beaten
50g (2 oz) sunflower margarine, melted
½ teaspoon crushed rosemary
freshly ground black pepper

1 Preheat the oven to 180°C/350°F/Gas 4.
2 Combine all the ingredients together and mix well. Press into a shallow 18cm (7 in) square cake tin.
3 Bake in the preheated oven for about 40 minutes until golden.
4 Cut into slices, and eat hot or cold.

Cornbread 123L *Makes 12 squares*

175g (6 oz) polenta
50g (2 oz) rice flour
50g (2 oz) potato flour
2–3 tablespoons unrefined brown sugar
2 teaspoons wheat-free baking powder
300ml (10 fl oz) tepid rice, soya or semi-skimmed milk
2 eggs, lightly beaten
50g (2 oz) sunflower margarine, melted and cooled slightly

1 Preheat the oven to 200°C/400°F/Gas 6, and lightly grease an 18cm (7 in) square cake tin.

2   Put the polenta, flours, sugar and baking powder into a large bowl and make a well in the middle. Pour in the milk, eggs and margarine, and beat the ingredients to form a batter.

3   Pour the mixture into the prepared cake tin and bake in the preheated oven for 25–30 minutes until golden.

4   Leave the cornbread to cool, then cut into squares. Serve warm or cold.

Variation

Chilli and Cheese Cornbread   (23L)

For a savoury variation to serve with Chilli con Carne, add to the cornbread mixture 225g (8 oz) grated Cheddar, and 1 cored, seeded and finely chopped green chilli, and follow method as above.

Cornmeal Muffins   123L   *Makes 12*

75g (3 oz) gram (chickpea) flour
100g (4 oz) cornmeal
1 tablespoon wheat-free baking powder
1 teaspoon sugar
1 teaspoon salt
275ml (9 fl oz) rice, soya or semi-skimmed milk
2 tablespoons corn oil
1 medium egg, beaten

1   Preheat the oven to 220°C/425°F/Gas 7, and lightly grease a 12-cup muffin tin or line with 12 paper cases.

2   Mix the flour, cornmeal, baking powder, sugar and salt together in a large bowl. Add the milk, oil and egg and

whisk together to make a smooth batter.

3   Spoon into the muffin cases and bake in the preheated oven for about 20 minutes until risen and pale golden brown. For the best taste, eat warm.

Potato Farls   123L   *Makes 12*

75g (3 oz) rice flour
75g (3 oz) potato flour
1 tablespoon wheat-free baking powder
50g (2 oz) sunflower margarine
45g (1½ oz) unrefined caster sugar
100g (4 oz) freshly boiled and mashed potato
3 tablespoons soya, rice or semi-skimmed milk

1   Preheat the oven to 220°C/425°F/Gas 7, and grease a baking tray.

2   Sift the flours and baking powder into a bowl. Rub in the sunflower margarine until the mixture resembles fine breadcrumbs. Stir in the sugar and mashed potato. Add enough milk to bind to a soft but not sticky dough.

3   Turn the dough on to a floured surface and knead lightly until blended. Roll out to 1cm (½ in) thick and cut into rectangles.

4   Place the rectangles on to the greased baking tray and bake in the preheated oven for 12–15 minutes until risen and golden.

5   Leave to cool on a wire rack. Serve the same day.

Potato and Rice Bread   123L   *Makes 2 loaves*

275g (10 oz) potato flour
225g (8 oz) brown rice flour
1½ packets easy-blend yeast
1 teaspoon unrefined caster sugar
1 tablespoon sunflower oil
½–1 teaspoon salt
300–350ml (10–12 fl oz) hand-hot water

1   Preheat the oven to 230°C/450°F/Gas 8, and grease and flour 2 × 450g (1 lb) loaf tins.

2   Mix together the flours and easy-blend yeast.

3   Add the sugar, oil and salt and mix to a thick batter with the hand-hot water.

4   Divide the mixture between the two prepared tins, cover and leave to rise in a warm place for 20–30 minutes.

5   Bake the loaves in the preheated oven for 35–40 minutes. The bread will slightly contract from the side of the tins when it is cooked.

6   Cool for 5 minutes in the tins and then turn on to a wire rack. Slice when cold.

Rice and Cornflour Crispbread   123L
Makes 12 squares or 8 'Ryvita' size shapes

100g (4 oz) brown rice flour
50g (2 oz) cornflour
2 tablespoons oil of your choice
warm water to mix

1 Preheat the oven to 220°C/425°F/Gas 7, and grease a baking tray.
2 Mix the flours and oil together. Add enough water to make a soft dough.
3 Roll the dough out thinly on a surface dusted with rice flour. Cut into oblong biscuits and place on a greased baking tray.
4 Bake in the preheated oven for 8–10 minutes. Leave to cool on a wire rack.

Sussex Rice and Corn Bread 123L

3 eggs
2 tablespoons unbleached brown sugar
3 tablespoons walnut oil
150g (5 oz) rice flour
150g (5 oz) cornflour
250ml (½ pint) milk
1 tablespoon water
1½ sachets fast-action dried yeast
½ teaspoon salt
2 heaped teaspoons wheat-free baking powder

This can be made using a breadmaker.

1 Place all the ingredients in a food processor or mixing bowl and beat until smooth.
2 Pour the mixture into the breadmaker and programme it for 3 hours.
3 Remove the cooked bread from the breadmaker and eat while warm or leave to cool.

4   Slice as conventional bread and serve with butter and pure
    fruit spread.

Note

- A four part combination of flour can be used
  (corn/rice/potato/soya) to give a total of 300g (10 oz).

- Linseeds and dried fruit can be added to the mixture
  (approximately 1 cup of mixed fruit and linseeds).

Beverages

Carrot and Apple Juice   123L   *Serves 2*

This is a drink rich in antioxidants; a good way to start the day.

6 large organic carrots, washed and scrubbed
2 eating apples of your choice, peeled and cored

Put the carrots and the apples through a juice extractor and
serve immediately.

Miss P's Punch   123L   *Makes 1 litre (1¾ pints)*

This makes a refreshing drink with or between meals, especially
served with ice on a hot day.

750ml (1¼ pints) water
200ml (7 fl oz) orange juice

3½ tablespoons blackcurrant concentrate (no added sugar)
2 yellow plums, chopped
2 red plums, chopped
1 orange, peeled, segmented and chopped
1 lemon, peeled and chopped
1 kiwi fruit, peeled and chopped
zest of 1 orange, peeled off in strips with a potato peeler or sharp
  knife

Mix all the ingredients together and serve chilled.

Watermelon and Ginger Juice   123L   *Serves 2*

This is a great 'pick-me-up' and also good for preventing headaches.

½ medium watermelon, seeded, skinned and chopped
25cm (1 in) square of fresh root ginger (adjust according to taste)
ice cubes

Put the ingredients through a juicer or blend in a liquidiser. Mix well and serve immediately.

ZFL Fruit Shake   123L   *Serves 2*

This mixture can be frozen in ice-cube trays to make fruity treats.

1 mango, stoned and peeled
½ honeydew melon, seeded, skinned and chopped
¼ pineapple, peeled and chopped

150ml (5 fl oz) fresh orange juice
ice cubes

Put the fruit through a juice extractor and mix with the orange juice. Add the ice cubes and serve.

ZFL Milkshake   123L   *Serves 1*

300ml (10 fl oz) appropriate milk for your stage (rice, soya or
*   semi-skimmed)*
1 banana
2 tablespoons ZFL sprinkle (see page 196)

Blend the ingredients together in a liquidiser and serve at once.

Part Four

Long-term Advice

Chapter 20

Zest for Life – A Life Plan

By the time you reach this final section of The Zest for Life Plan you should be looking good, feeling well and proud of your achievement. The general consensus is that the voyage through this plan is a learning curve through previously untrodden territory. Now that you know how to interpret your body's messages and have become familiar with what it likes and dislikes, you will no doubt agree with many of the following points.

- That the process was not terribly difficult and worth the effort involved.

- The knowledge you have gleaned whilst reading should have been available to you earlier in life.

- Your diet and lifestyle have a tremendous effect on both your physical and mental well-being.

- Ideally we, the consumers, should have more control over the food we eat.

- Our food labels should reveal the precise contents of food, and the chemical processes it has been subjected to.

You may feel more involved now with food issues. I am sure that the organisations would appreciate your help and support – you can find details on page 357.

Formulating your long-term plan

You will probably be only too aware of any reactions experienced during the three stages of ZFL, but it is still worth setting a little time aside both to review your progress and make a plan for the future.

- As you look through the weekly charts you will have made, make a list of any foods or drinks that definitely seemed to cause a reaction, which will be known as your 'black list'. Another list of items that you are currently unsure of will be your 'grey list'.

- What you need to concentrate on is all the products on your 'white list' (the foods and drinks you seemed to thrive on) for the next few weeks, taking care to omit items on both the grey and black lists from your diet.

- When you feel the time is right, for example, when you are feeling really well, or when you have reached and maintained your target weight for a few months, re-test the grey list by introducing them back into your diet one by one. As before, leave five days between foods.

- Another few months down the line, re-test the remaining foods on the grey list gradually, one by one as before. Sometimes when the body is in better nutritional shape the tolerance to certain foods and drinks improves.

- The foods and drinks that remain on both the grey list and the black list may be tested again several months down the line, but always individually, leaving plenty of time for any reaction to reveal itself.

Continuing the plan

If you had a considerable amount of weight to lose, and have not achieved your target weight by the end of The Zest for Life Plan, there is nothing to stop you continuing for as many months as you wish. Unlike other weight-loss diets, ZFL is designed to be followed in the long term because, as you will have gathered by now, ZFL provides you with all the important nutrients your body needs in order to thrive.

Neither is there any need for you to revert to your old way of eating when you have completed ZFL. It will be much better for your health and well-being in the long term if you remain on the regime, perhaps increasing the portion sizes a little, or adding in some of the little long-term treats listed in the dessert section, for example. There is no harm in deviating from your basic diet on special occasions or at holiday times, as you are now armed with the knowledge of what your body really needs on a regular basis. And we firmly believe that, when you are well, 'a little of what you fancy does you good'.

What about introducing wheat?

If weight loss has been your main motivation for following ZFL, be wary about introducing wheat before you have reached your target weight. In our experience, many people who are not in brilliant nutritional shape, and whose immune systems may not be operating in an optimal fashion, may retain fluid as part of an adverse chemical reaction to wholewheat or bran. It is therefore advisable to leave the reintroduction of wholewheat or wheat bran until you have achieved your target weight, and have overcome any bowel symptoms or fatigue, if they were part of your 'baggage'.

Once you are feeling well and have lost the desired weight, feel free to reintroduce wholewheat products gradually over a period of a week or two, whilst keeping careful notes of any symptoms that may occur and watching your weight like a hawk. If the scales show that the pounds are creeping back on – beware. It may be that at this point you can tolerate wheat in small quantities, which will mean that you can eat it 'socially' rather than as part of your everyday diet.

If the reaction to wheat is severe, it is best to exclude it completely from your diet for at least the next few months, before having another attempt at its reintroduction. You will have discovered by now that there are plenty of delicious alternatives freely available, and it may even be that you are quite happy with your current diet, and stopped pining for wheat some time ago.

What about alcohol in the long term?

Once you have completed The Zest for Life Plan and are feeling happy with your weight, you can reintroduce alcohol gradually. Ideally, begin with just an occasional drink, noting any adverse side-effects if they occur. If you manage to maintain your well-being and consume alcohol, you can continue to increase the number of drinks until you reach approximately 7 units per week (1 unit = 1 glass of wine, 300ml (½ pint) lager or beer, or 1 measure of spirit). The maximum acceptable number of units per week is 14 for women, 21 for men, but as alcohol tends to knock most nutrients sideways as well as being rich in calories, it may be advisable to drink alcohol in moderation, except on high days and holidays.

If you feel the worse for wear after drinking, it will be better to refrain for a while so that your body can recover. If you do experience a reaction, bear in mind that grape and grain may produce different effects. Those continuing to avoid wheat should also avoid beer and lager as they are grain products. Wine, gin and vodka may be acceptable as they are made from fruit and vegetables. I have had patients who, although they could not tolerate ordinary wine, found they felt fine after drinking organic wine. Sometimes the chemicals contained in wine can make us feel worse than the alcohol itself.

When reintroducing alcohol, as with any other group of foods or drinks, maintain your weekly record charts; if you happen to experience symptoms, these charts will help you to detect the cause.

Supplements for the long term

At the WNAS we do not recommend long-term pill-popping, but we do recognise that there are times when supplements will improve the quality of life, especially when taken in reduced doses over a period of time. The supplements that may be required during the various phases of life will vary, as you will have gathered from reading chapter 11, and during ZFL you will have had the opportunity to experiment with supplements that you felt were indicated. As we are all so different, your long-term supplement programme, should you decide that supplements are necessary, will be the result of trial and error over the months, until you find the regime that seems to suit you. There will be times when you need to change your regime – for example when you are actively planning to conceive, are pregnant or breastfeeding, or moving from your childbearing years into the menopause. I suggest you read our book, *Every Woman's Health Guide*, which outlines 120 different conditions, and contains full details about both what your doctor has to offer, and what you can do to help yourself.

Keep fit and make time for yourself

Unfortunately, most of us have to work at remaining in good physical and mental shape. Whilst it may take a while and some in-depth personal persuasion to get a regular exercise programme established, I think you will agree that it gives you a regular infusion of that 'feel-good factor'. So don't get complacent at the end of ZFL and think you feel so well there is no need to continue. Many have made that mistake before and lived to regret it! Enjoy your exercise regime, and make time to relax on a regular basis, even if it's only for fifteen minutes per day. We all need time to reflect on our lives, on decisions that need to be made, and indeed on our achievements. The time you invest in exercise and relaxation will be repaid many times in terms of increased energy and elevated mood. When you feel positive, happy and energetic, you are bound to achieve more in life, and to attract more interesting company.

Having shown tens of thousands of women how to help themselves to better health over the last fourteen years, I really believe that in the final analysis it is up to each individual to invest in themselves. Once armed with the knowledge, which of course you now are, the quality of your health in the long term is very much in your own hands. You may regard this as a somewhat daunting prospect, but it very definitely puts you in the driving seat. The only side-effects you are likely to experience are that you will be looking good and feeling fine for a long time to come!

Appendix I

Weekly Diary and Review

ZFL WEEKLY DIARY

DATE:

PLEASE COMPLETE THE DIARY ON A DAILY BASIS AND GRADE SYMPTOMS ON A SCALE OF 0–3 ACCORDING TO SEVERITY WITH:

0 = NONE, 1 = MILD, 2 = MODERATE, 3 = SEVERE

	BREAKFAST	LUNCH	DINNER	SNACKS	EXERCISE	SUPPLEMENTS	RELAXATION	SYMPTOMS	REACTIONS
DAY 1									
DAY 2									
DAY 3									
DAY 4									
DAY 5									
DAY 6									
DAY 7									

ZFL WEEKLY DIARY

DATE:

PLEASE COMPLETE THE DIARY ON A DAILY BASIS AND GRADE SYMPTOMS ON A SCALE OF 0–3 ACCORDING TO SEVERITY WITH:

0 = NONE, 1 = MILD, 2 = MODERATE, 3 = SEVERE

	BREAKFAST	LUNCH	DINNER	SNACKS	EXERCISE	SUPPLEMENTS	RELAXATION	SYMPTOMS	REACTIONS
DAY 1									
DAY 2									
DAY 3									
DAY 4									
DAY 5									
DAY 6									
DAY 7									

ZFL WEEKLY DIARY

DATE:

PLEASE COMPLETE THE DIARY ON A DAILY BASIS AND GRADE SYMPTOMS ON A SCALE OF 0–3 ACCORDING TO SEVERITY WITH:

0 = NONE, 1 = MILD, 2 = MODERATE, 3 = SEVERE

	BREAKFAST	LUNCH	DINNER	SNACKS	EXERCISE	SUPPLEMENTS	RELAXATION	SYMPTOMS	REACTIONS
DAY 1									
DAY 2									
DAY 3									
DAY 4									
DAY 5									
DAY 6									
DAY 7									

ZFL REVIEW

WHITE LIST = Foods and drinks that you seem well on
GREY LIST =   Foods and drinks that you are unsure of currently
BLACK LIST = Foods and drinks you had a reaction to

STAGE I	WHITE LIST	GREY LIST	BLACK LIST

STAGE II	WHITE LIST	GREY LIST	BLACK LIST

STAGE III	WHITE LIST	GREY LIST	BLACK LIST

Appendix II

Nutritional Content of Food Lists

Foods containing **Vitamin A – Retinol** (Micrograms per 100 g/3.5 oz)

mcg		mcg	
1	Skimmed milk	325	Cheddar cheese
21	Semi-skimmed milk	800	Margarine
49	Grilled herring	815	Butter
52	Whole milk	15,000	Lamb's liver
56	Porridge made with milk		

Foods containing **Vitamin B1 – Thiamin** (Milligrams per 100 g/3.5 oz)

mg		mg	
0.02	Peaches	0.10	Oranges
0.02	Cottage cheese	0.10	Brussels sprouts
0.03	Cox's apple	0.11	Potatoes, new, boiled
0.04	Full-fat milk	0.12	Soya beans, boiled
0.04	Skimmed milk	0.12	Red peppers, raw
0.04	Semi-skimmed milk	0.14	Lentils, boiled
0.04	Cheddar cheese	0.20	Steamed salmon
0.04	Bananas	0.20	Corn
0.04	White grapes	0.21	White spaghetti, boiled
0.04	French beans	0.24	Almonds
0.05	Low-fat yoghurt	0.30	White self-raising flour
0.05	Cantaloupe melon	0.30	Plaice, steamed
0.06	Tomato	0.35	Bacon, cooked
0.07	Green peppers, raw	0.40	Walnuts
0.08	Boiled egg	0.47	Wholemeal flour
0.08	Roast chicken	0.49	Lamb's kidney
0.08	Grilled cod	1.00	Brazil nuts
0.08	Haddock, steamed	1.00	Cornflakes
0.09	Roast turkey	1.00	Rice Krispies
0.09	Mackerel, cooked	2.01	Wheatgerm
0.10	Savoy cabbage, boiled		

Foods containing **Vitamin B2 – Riboflavin** (Milligrams per 100 g/3.5 oz)

mg		mg	
0.01	Cabbage, boiled	0.11	Baked salmon
0.01	Potatoes, boiled	0.15	Red peppers, raw
0.02	Brown rice, boiled	0.17	Full-fat milk
0.03	Pear	0.18	Avocado
	Wholemeal spaghetti,	0.18	Grilled herring
0.03	boiled	0.18	Semi-skimmed milk
0.03	White self-raising flour	0.19	Roast chicken
0.04	Orange	0.21	Roast turkey
	Spinach, boiled in salted	0.26	Cottage cheese
0.05	water	0.31	Soya flour
0.06	Baked beans	0.34	Boiled prawns
0.06	Banana	0.35	Boiled egg
0.06	White bread	0.35	Topside of beef, cooked
0.08	Green peppers, raw	0.38	Leg of lamb, cooked
0.08	Lentils, boiled	0.40	Cheddar cheese
0.09	Hovis	0.70	Muesli
0.09	Soya beans, boiled	0.75	Almonds
0.09	Wholemeal bread	1.50	Cornflakes
0.09	Wholemeal flour	1.50	Rice Krispies
0.10	Peanuts		

Foods containing **Vitamin B3 – Niacin** (Milligrams per 100 g/3.5 oz)

mg		mg	
0.07	Boiled egg	1.50	White self-raising flour
0.07	Cheddar cheese	1.70	Grilled cod
0.08	Full-fat milk	1.70	White bread
0.09	Skimmed milk	2.00	Soya flour
0.09	Semi-skimmed milk	2.20	Red peppers, raw
0.13	Cottage cheese	3.10	Almonds
0.20	Cox's apple	4.00	Grilled herring
0.30	Cabbage, boiled	4.10	Wholemeal bread
0.40	Orange	4.20	Hovis
0.50	Baked beans	5.70	Wholemeal flour
0.50	Potatoes, boiled	6.50	Muesli
0.50	Soya beans, boiled	6.50	Topside of beef, cooked
0.60	Lentils, boiled	6.60	Leg of lamb, cooked
0.70	Banana	7.00	Baked salmon
1.00	Tomato	8.20	Roast chicken
1.10	Avocado	8.50	Roast turkey
1.10	Green peppers, raw	9.50	Boiled prawns
1.30	Brown rice	13.80	Peanuts
	Wholemeal	16.00	Cornflakes
1.30	spaghetti,boiled	16.00	Rice Krispies

Foods containing **Vitamin B6 – Pyridoxine** (Milligrams per 100 g/3.5 oz)

mg		mg	
0.05	Carrots	0.19	Brussels sprouts
0.06	Full-fat milk	0.21	Sweetcorn, boiled
0.06	Skimmed milk	0.22	Leg of lamb, cooked
0.06	Semi-skimmed milk	0.23	Grapefruit juice
0.07	Satsuma	0.26	Roast chicken
0.07	White bread	0.28	Lentils, boiled
0.07	White rice	0.29	Banana
0.08	Cabbage, boiled	0.31	Brazil nuts
0.08	Cottage cheese	0.32	Potatoes, boiled
0.08	Cox's apple	0.33	Roast turkey
0.08	Wholemeal pasta	0.33	Grilled herring
0.09	Frozen peas	0.33	Topside of beef, cooked
0.09	Spinach, boiled	0.36	Avocado
0.10	Cheddar cheese	0.38	Grilled cod
0.10	Orange	0.57	Baked salmon
0.11	Broccoli	0.57	Soya flour
0.11	Hovis	0.59	Hazelnuts
0.12	Baked beans	0.59	Peanuts
0.12	Boiled egg	0.67	Walnuts
0.12	Red kidney beans, cooked	1.60	Muesli
0.12	Wholemeal bread	1.80	Cornflakes
0.14	Tomatoes	1.80	Rice Krispies
0.15	Almonds	2.20	Special K
0.15	Cauliflower		

Foods containing **Vitamin B12** (Micrograms per 100 g/3.5 oz)

mcg		mcg	
0.10	Tempeh	2.00	Rice Krispies
0.20	Miso	2.00	Steak, lean, grilled
0.30	Quorn	2.10	Edam cheese
0.40	Full-fat milk	2.40	Eggs, whole, battery
0.40	Skimmed milk	2.40	Milk, dried, whole
0.40	Semi-skimmed milk	2.60	Milk, dried, skimmed
0.50	Marmite	2.70	Eggs, whole, free-range
0.70	Cottage cheese	2.80	Kambu seaweed
1.00	Choux buns	2.90	Squid, frozen
1.00	Eggs, boiled	2.90	Taramasalata
1.00	Eggs, poached	3.00	Duck, cooked
1.00	Halibut, steamed	3.00	Turkey, dark meat
1.00	Lobster, boiled	5.00	Grapenuts
1.00	Sponge cake	5.00	Tuna in oil
1.00	Turkey, white meat	6.00	Herring, cooked
1.00	Waffles	6.00	Herring roe, fried
1.20	Cheddar cheese	6.00	Steamed salmon
1.20	Eggs, scrambled	8.30	Bovril
1.30	Squid	10.00	Mackerel, fried
1.60	Eggs, fried	10.00	Rabbit, stewed
1.80	Shrimps, boiled	11.00	Cod's roe, fried
1.90	Parmesan cheese		Pilchards canned in
2.00	Beef, lean	12.00	tomato juice
2.00	Cod, baked	15.00	Oysters, raw
2.00	Cornflakes	27.50	Nori seaweed
2.00	Pork, cooked	28.00	Sardines in oil
2.00	Raw beef mince	79.00	Lamb's kidney, fried

Foods containing **Folate/Folic acid** (Micrograms per 100 g/3.5 oz)

mcg		mcg	
4.00	Cox's apple	31.00	Orange
4.00	Leg of lamb, cooked	33.00	Baked beans
6.00	Full-fat milk	33.00	Cheddar cheese
6.00	Skimmed milk	33.00	Clementines
6.00	Semi-skimmed milk	33.00	Raspberries
	Porridge with	33.00	Satsuma
7.00	semi-skimmed milk	34.00	Blackberries
8.00	Turnip, baked	35.00	Rye crispbread
8.00	Sweet potato, boiled	36.00	Potato, baked in skin
9.00	Cucumber	38.00	Radish
10.00	Grilled herring	39.00	Boiled egg
10.00	Roast chicken	39.00	Hovis
11.00	Avocado	39.00	Wholemeal bread
12.00	Grilled cod	42.00	Red kidney beans, boiled
14.00	Banana	44.00	Potato, baked
15.00	Roast turkey	47.00	Frozen peas
17.00	Carrots	48.00	Almonds
17.00	Sweet potato	48.00	Parsnips, boiled
17.00	Tomatoes	51.00	Cauliflower
17.00	Topside of beef, cooked	57.00	Green beans, boiled
18.00	Swede, boiled	64.00	Broccoli
20.00	Strawberries	66.00	Walnuts
21.00	Brazil nuts	68.00	Artichoke
21.00	Red peppers, raw	72.00	Hazelnuts
23.00	Green peppers, raw	90.00	Spinach, boiled
24.00	Rye bread	110.00	Brussels sprouts
25.00	Dates, fresh	110.00	Peanuts
25.00	New potatoes, boiled	140.00	Muesli
26.00	Grapefruit	150.00	Sweetcorn, boiled
26.00	Oatcakes	155.00	Asparagus
27.00	Cottage cheese	180.00	Chickpeas
29.00	Baked salmon	240.00	Lamb's liver, fried
29.00	Cabbage, boiled	250.00	Cornflakes
29.00	Onions, boiled	250.00	Rice Krispies
29.00	White bread	320.00	Calf's liver, fried

Foods containing **Vitamin C** (Milligrams per 100 g/3.5 oz)

mg		mg	
1.00	Full-fat milk	17.00	Melon
1.00	Skimmed milk	17.00	Tomatoes
1.00	Semi-skimmed milk	20.00	Cabbage, boiled
1.00	Red kidney beans	26.00	Canteloupe melon
2.00	Carrots	27.00	Cauliflower
2.00	Cucumber	27.00	Satsuma
2.00	Muesli with dried fruit	31.00	Peach
6.00	Apricots, raw	32.00	Raspberries
6.00	Avocado	35.00	Bran flakes
6.00	Pear	36.00	Grapefruit
6.00	Potato, boiled	37.00	Mangoes
8.00	Spinach, boiled	37.00	Nectarine
9.00	Cox's apple	39.00	Kumquats
10.00	Turnip	44.00	Broccoli
11.00	Banana	45.00	Lychees
12.00	Frozen peas	49.00	Unsweetened apple juice
12.00	Lamb's liver, fried	54.00	Orange
12.00	Pineapple	59.00	Kiwi fruit
13.00	Dried skimmed milk	60.00	Brussels sprouts
14.00	Gooseberries	77.00	Strawberries
14.00	Raw dates	115.00	Blackcurrants

Foods containing **Vitamin D** (Micrograms per 100 g/3.5 oz)

mcg		mcg	
0.01	Skimmed milk	2.80	Cornflakes
0.03	Whole milk	2.80	Rice Krispies
0.05	Fromage frais	4.20	Kellogg's Start
0.26	Cheddar cheese	8.00	Margarine

Foods containing **Vitamin E** (Milligrams per 100 g/3.5 oz)

mg		mg	
0.03	Semi-skimmed milk		Unsweetened orange
0.06	Boiled potatoes	0.68	juice
0.07	Cucumber	0.78	Leeks
0.08	Cottage cheese	0.88	Sweetcorn, boiled
0.09	Full-fat milk	0.90	Brussels sprouts
0.10	Cabbage, boiled	1.10	Broccoli
0.10	Leg of lamb, cooked	1.11	Boiled egg
0.11	Cauliflower	1.22	Tomato
0.11	Roast chicken	1.46	Watercress
0.18	Frozen peas	1.70	Parsley
	Red kidney beans,	1.71	Spinach, boiled
0.20	cooked	1.99	Olives
0.20	Wholemeal bread	2.00	Butter
0.24	Orange	2.69	Onions, dried raw
0.26	Topside of beef, cooked		Mushrooms, fried in corn
0.27	Banana	2.84	oil
0.30	Brown rice, boiled	3.20	Avocado
0.30	Grilled herring	3.20	Muesli
0.32	Lamb's liver, fried	3.85	Walnuts
0.36	Baked beans	4.99	Peanut butter
0.40	Cornflakes	5.10	Olive oil
0.50	Pear	5.96	Sweet potato, baked
0.53	Cheddar cheese	7.18	Brazil nuts
0.56	Carrots	10.09	Peanuts
0.57	Lettuce	13.65	Pine nuts
0.59	Cox's apple	18.40	Rapeseed oil
0.59	Grilled cod	23.96	Almonds
0.60	Rice Krispies	24.98	Hazelnuts
0.61	Plums	48.70	Sunflower oil

Foods containing **Calcium** (Milligrams per 100 g/3.5 oz)

mg		mg	
4.00	Cox's apple	47.00	Orange
4.00	Brown rice, boiled	48.00	Baked beans
5.00	Potatoes, boiled	54.00	Wholemeal bread
6.00	Banana	57.00	Boiled egg
6.00	Topside of beef, cooked	60.00	Peanuts
7.00	White pasta, boiled	73.00	Cottage cheese
7.00	Tomato	83.00	Soya beans, boiled
7.00	White spaghetti, boiled	100.00	White bread
8.00	Leg of lamb, cooked	115.00	Full-fat milk
8.00	Red peppers, raw	120.00	Hovis
9.00	Roast chicken	120.00	Muesli
9.00	Roast turkey	120.00	Skimmed milk
11.00	Avocado	120.00	Semi-skimmed milk
11.00	Pear	150.00	Prawns, boiled
15.00	Butter	150.00	Spinach, boiled
15.00	Cornflakes	170.00	Brazil nuts
18.00	White rice, boiled	190.00	Yoghurt, low-fat, plain
22.00	Grilled cod	210.00	Soya flour
22.00	Lentils, boiled	240.00	Almonds
29.00	Baked salmon	450.00	White self-raising flour
30.00	Green peppers, raw	550.00	Sardines
30.00	Young carrots	710.00	Sprats, fried
33.00	Grilled herring	720.00	Cheddar cheese
38.00	Wholemeal flour	860.00	Whitebait, fried
45.00	Turnips, baked		

Foods containing **Chromium** (Micrograms per 100 g/3.5 oz)

mcg		mcg	
183.00	Egg yolk	56.00	Hard cheese
121.00	Molasses	55.00	Liver
117.00	Brewer's yeast	47.00	Fruit juices
57.00	Beef	42.00	Wholemeal bread

Foods containing **Iron** (Milligrams per 100 g/3.5 oz)

mg		mg	
0.05	Semi-skimmed milk	1.10	Boiled prawns
0.06	Skimmed milk	1.20	Green peppers, raw
0.06	Full-fat milk	1.40	Baked beans
0.10	Cottage cheese		Wholemeal spaghetti,
0.10	Orange	1.40	boiled
0.20	Cox's apple	1.60	White bread
0.20	Pear	1.70	Spinach, boiled
0.20	White rice	1.90	Boiled egg
0.30	Banana	2.00	White self-raising flour
0.30	Cabbage, boiled	2.50	Brazil nuts
0.30	Cheddar cheese	2.50	Peanuts
0.40	Avocado	2.70	Leg of lamb, cooked
0.40	Grilled cod	2.70	Wholemeal bread
0.40	Potatoes, boiled	2.80	Topside of beef, cooked
0.40	Young carrots, boiled	3.00	Almonds
0.50	Brown rice, boiled	3.00	Soya beans, boiled
0.50	Tomato	3.50	Lentils, boiled
0.50	White pasta, boiled	3.70	Hovis
0.80	Baked salmon	3.90	Wholemeal flour
0.80	Roast chicken	5.60	Muesli
0.90	Roast turkey	6.70	Cornflakes
1.00	Grilled herring	6.70	Rice Krispies
1.00	Red peppers, raw	6.90	Soya flour

Foods containing **Magnesium** (Milligrams per 100 g/3.5 oz)

mg		mg	
2.00	Butter	26.00	Grilled cod
6.00	Cox's apple	27.00	Roast turkey
6.00	Turnip, baked	28.00	Leg of lamb, cooked
6.00	Young carrots	29.00	Baked salmon
7.00	Tomato	31.00	Baked beans
9.00	Cottage cheese	31.00	Spinach, boiled
10.00	Orange	32.00	Grilled herring
11.00	Full-fat milk	34.00	Banana
11.00	White rice, boiled	34.00	Lentils, boiled
11.00	Semi-skimmed milk	42.00	Boiled prawns
12.00	Skimmed milk		Wholemeal spaghetti,
12.00	Boiled egg	42.00	boiled
14.00	Cornflakes	43.00	Brown rice, boiled
14.00	Potatoes, boiled	56.00	Hovis
14.00	Red peppers, raw	63.00	Soya beans, boiled
15.00	White pasta	76.00	Wholemeal bread
20.00	White self-raising flour	85.00	Muesli
24.00	Green peppers, raw	120.00	Wholemeal flour
24.00	Roast chicken	210.00	Peanuts
24.00	Topside of beef, cooked	240.00	Soya flour
24.00	White bread	270.00	Almonds
25.00	Avocado	410.00	Brazil nuts
25.00	Cheddar cheese		

Foods containing **Selenium** (Micrograms per 100 g/3.5 oz)

mcg		mcg	
1.00	Full-fat milk	4.00	White rice
1.00	Semi-skimmed milk	4.00	White self-raising flour
1.00	Skimmed milk	5.00	Soya beans, boiled
2.00	Baked beans	11.00	Boiled egg
2.00	Cornflakes	12.00	Cheddar cheese
2.00	Orange	28.00	White bread
3.00	Peanuts	35.00	Wholemeal bread
4.00	Almonds	40.00	Lentils, boiled
4.00	Cottage cheese	53.00	Wholemeal flour

Foods containing **Zinc** (Milligrams per 100 g/3.5 oz)

mg		mg	
0.10	Butter	0.60	White self-raising flour
0.10	Pear	0.70	Brown rice
0.10	Orange	0.70	White rice
0.10	Red peppers, raw	0.90	Soya beans, boiled
0.20	Banana		Wholemeal spaghetti,
0.20	Young carrots	1.10	boiled
0.30	Cornflakes	1.30	Boiled egg
0.30	Potatoes, boiled	1.40	Lentils, boiled
0.40	Avocado	1.50	Roast chicken
0.40	Full-fat milk	1.60	Boiled prawns
0.40	Skimmed milk	1.80	Wholemeal bread
0.40	Green peppers, raw	2.10	Hovis
0.40	Semi-skimmed milk	2.30	Cheddar cheese
0.50	Baked beans	2.40	Roast turkey
0.50	Grilled cod	2.50	Muesli
0.50	Grilled herring	2.90	Wholemeal flour
0.50	White pasta	3.20	Almonds
0.50	Tomatoes	3.50	Peanuts
0.60	Cottage cheese	4.20	Brazil nuts
0.60	Spinach, boiled	5.30	Leg of lamb, cooked
0.60	White bread	5.50	Topside of beef, cooked

Foods containing **Essential fatty acids**

Exact amounts of these fats are hard to quantify. Good sources for the two families of essential fatty acids are given.

Omega 6 Series Essential Fatty Acids

Sunflower oil
Rapeseed oil
Corn oil
Almonds
Walnuts
Brazil nuts
Sunflower seeds
Soya products including tofu

Omega 3 Series Essential Fatty Acids

Mackerel
Herring   } fresh cooked or smoked/pickled
Salmon
Walnuts and walnut oil
Rapeseed oil
Soya products and soya oil

Suggested Reading List

UK, USA and Aus denote the following books are available in Great Britain, United States of America and Australia.

Diet

The Allergy Diet by Elizabeth Workman SRD, Dr John Hunter and Dr Virginia Alun Jones. Published by Martin Dunitz. UK, USA.

Food Allergy and Intolerance by Jonathan Brostoff and Linda Gamlin. Published by Bloomsbury. UK, Aus.

The Real Food Shop and Restaurant Guide by Clive Johnstone. Published by Ebury Press. UK.

Beat Sugar Craving by Maryon Stewart. Published by Vermilion (available from Nutritional Health Limited). UK.

Organic Consumer Guide/Food You Can Trust edited by David Mabey and Alan and Jackie Gear. Published by Thorsons. UK.

The New Raw Energy by Leslie and Susannah Kenton. Published by Vermilion. UK, Aus.

Foresight Index Number Decoder (Packet Additive Dictionary) available from Foresight. UK.

What the Label Doesn't Tell You by Sue Dibb (available from the Food Commission). UK.

Recipe books

Good Food Gluten Free by Hilda Cherry Hills. Published by Keats. USA.

Gluten-free Cookery by Rita Greer. Published by Thorsons. UK.

The Wheat and Gluten Free Cookbook by Joan Noble. Published by Vermilion. UK, Aus.

The Candida Albicans Yeast-free Cook Book by Pat Connolly and Associates of the Price Pottenger Nutrition Foundation. Published by Keats. UK, USA.

The Cranks Recipe Book by David Canter, Hay Canter and Daphne Swann. Published by Orion. UK.

Raw Energy Recipes by Leslie and Susannah Kenton. Published by Century. UK.

The Reluctant Vegetarian Cook by Simon Hope. Published by Heinemann. UK.

Gourmet Vegetarian Cooking by Rose Elliot. Published by Fontana. UK, Aus.

The Gluten-free and Wheat-free Bumper Bake Book by Rita Greer. Published by Bunterbird Ltd. UK.

The Single Vegan by Leah Leneman. Published by Thorsons. UK.

Whole Earth Cookbook by Hilary Meth. Published by Vermilion. UK

Beat PMS Cookbook by Maryon Stewart and Sarah Tooley. Published by Vermilion and available from Nutritional Health Limited. UK.

General health

Every Woman's Health Guide by Maryon Stewart and Dr Alan Stewart. Published by Headline. UK, Aus.

Healthy Parents, Healthy Baby by Maryon Stewart and Dr Alan Stewart. Published by Headline. UK.

Nutritional Medicine by Dr Stephen Davies and Dr Alan Stewart. Published by Pan Books, UK.

Pure White and Deadly by Professor John Yudkin. Published by Viking. UK, Aus.

Food Allergy and Intolerance by Jonathan Brostoff and Linda Gamlin. Published by Bloomsbury. UK, Aus.

Tired All the Time by Dr Alan Stewart. Published by Vermilion. UK, USA, Aus.

No More IBS by Maryon Stewart and Dr Alan Stewart. Published by Vermilion. UK, Aus.

Beat the Menopause without HRT by Maryon Stewart. Published by Headline. UK.

No More PMS by Maryon Stewart. Published by Vermilion. UK.

Candida – Diet Against It by Luc de Schepper. Published by Foulsham. UK.

Exercise (Video)

Diana Moran's 3 in 1 Workout Video by Diana Moran. UK.

The Ys Way to Physical Fitness by Clayton R Myers and Lawrence A Golding (available from the YMCA). UK.

YMCA Guide to Exercise to Music by Rodney Cullum and Lesley Mowbray (available from the YMCA). UK.

Appendix IV

Useful Addresses

Alcoholics Anonymous (AA)
General Services Office, PO Box 1, Stonebow House, Stonebow, York YO1 2NJ. Tel: 01904 644026.

ASH (Campaign for Freedom from Tobacco)
Devon House, 12–15 Dartmouth Street, London SW1H 9BL. Tel: 0171 314 1360.

British Acupuncture Register and Directory
34 Alderney Street, London SW1V 4EU. Tel: 0171 834 1012

British Association for Counselling
1 Regent Place, Rugby, Warwickshire CV21 2PJ. Tel: 01788 578328 (info).

British College for Naturopathy and Osteopathy
6 Netherhall Gardens, London NW3 5RR. Tel: 0171 435 6464.

The British Homeopathic Association
27a Devonshire Street, London W1N 1RJ. Tel: 0171 935 2163.

British School of Osteopathy
1–4 Suffolk Street, London SW1Y 4HG. Tel: 0171 930 9254.

British Wheel of Yoga
1 Hamilton Place, Boston Road, Sleaford, Lincolnshire NG34 7ES. Tel: 01529 306851.

Depression Alliance
PO Box 1022, London SE1 7QB. Tel: 0171 721 7672.

Eating Disorders Association
Sackville Place, 44 Magdalen Street, Norwich NR3 1JU. Tel: 01603 621414.

The European School of Osteopathy
104 Tonbridge Road, Maidstone, Kent ME16 8SL. Tel: 01622 671558.

Exercise Association
4 Angel Gate, City Road, London EC1V 2PT. Tel: 0171 278 0811.

FLAG
Stephanie Cargill, PO Box 105, Hampton, Middlesex TW12 3TL. Tel: 0181 941 2977.

The Food Commission
94 White Lion Street, London N1 9PF. Tel: 0171 837 2250.

Foresight
28 The Paddock, Godalming, Surrey GU7 1XD.

Friends of the Earth
26–28 Underwood Street, London N1 7JQ. Tel: 0171 490 1555.

The Henry Doubleday Research Association
Ryton Gardens, National Centre for Organic Gardening, Ryton on Dunsmore, Coventry CV8 3LG. Tel: 01203 303517.

Migraine Trust
45 Great Ormond Street, London WC1N 3HZ. Tel: 0171 278 2676.

The National Institute of Medical Herbalists
56 Longbrook Street, Exeter EX4 6AN. Tel: 01392 426022.

The National Osteoporosis Society
Barton Meade House, PO Box 10, Radstock, Bath BA3 3YB

National Society for Research into Allergy
PO Box 45, Hinkley, Leicestershire LE10 1JY. Tel: 01455 851546.

Patients' Association
8 Guildford Street, London WC1N 1DT. Tel: 0171 242 3460.

The Samaritans
10 The Grove, Slough, SL1 1QP. Tel: 01753 532713.

School of Phytotherapy (Herbal Medicine)
Bucksteep Manor, Bodle Street Green, Nr Hailsham BN27 4RJ. Tel: 01323 833812/4.

The Shiatsu Society
31 Pullman Lane, Godalming, Surrey GU7 1XY. Tel: 01272 290661.

The Sports Council
16 Upper Woburn Place, London WC1H 0QP. Tel: 0171 388
1277.

Trax (UK) Ltd
National Tranquilliser Advice Centre, 25a Masons Avenue,
Wealdstone, Harrow, Middlesex HA3 5AH. Tel: (client line)
0181 427 2065 (24 hr answering service 0181 427 2827).

UK Action Against Allergy
PO Box 278, Twickenham TW1 42Q.

Vegan Society
Donald Watson House, 7 Battle Road, St Leonards on Sea,
East Sussex TN3Y 7AA. Tel: 01424 427393.

Vegetarian Society
Parkdale, Dunham Road, Altrincham, Cheshire WA14 4QG.
Tel: 0161 928 0793.

Women's Nutritional Advisory Service
PO Box 268, Lewes, East Sussex BN7 2QN. Tel: 01273
487366.

YMCA
112 Great Russell Street, London WC1B 3NQ. Tel: 0171 637
8131.

Australia

Adelaide Women's Community Health
64 Pennington Terrace, Nth Adelaide SA 5006. Tel: 08 267
5366.

Blackmores Limited – Women's Health Advisory Service
23 Roseberry Street, PO Box 258, Balgowlah, NSW 2093.
Tel: 00612 951 0111.

Liverpool Women's Health Centre
26 Bathurst Street, Liverpool NSW 2170. Tel: 02 601 3555.

Women's Health Advisory Service
155 Eaglecreek Road, Werombi, NSW 2570. Tel: 046 531
445.

New Zealand

Health Alternative for Women
Room 101, Cranmer Centre, PO Box 884, Christchurch. Tel:
796 970.

Papakura Women's Centre
4 Opaneke Road, Papakura, Auckland. Tel: 08267 5366.

Tauranga Women's Centre
PO Box 368, Tauranga. Tel: 075 783 530.

West Auckland Women's Centre
PO Box 69116, Glendene, Auckland. Tel: 09 838 6381.

Women's Health Collective
63 Ponsonby Road, Ponsonby, Auckland. Tel: 764 506.

Appendix V

Further Help and Telephone Advice Lines

If you would like to attend one of the WNAS clinics or need further details about our telephone and postal courses of treatment, you can write to the WNAS at the address below with an A5 self-addressed envelope and four separate first-class stamps. Please state clearly what information you require, e.g. general health/weight loss/fatigue/PMS/menopause/IBS, etc.

I should also be interested to hear about your success using the recommendations in this book.

The address to write to is:

Women's Nutritional Advisory Service
PO Box 268, Lewes, East Sussex BN7 2QN

All clinic appointments are booked on 01273 487366. Our mail order service for supplements and books is also on this number.

In addition we have a number of advice lines you may be interested in listening to:

0839 556602   Overcome Menopause Naturally

0839 556603   The Menopause Diet Line

0839 556600   Overcome PMS Naturally

0839 556601   The PMS Diet Line

0839 556604   Beat Sugar Craving

0839 556605   The Vitality Diet Line

0839 556606   Overcoming Breast Tenderness

0839 556607   Overcome Period Pains Naturally

0839 556608   Get Fit for Pregnancy and Breastfeeding

0839 556609   Skin, Nail & Hair Signs of Deficiency

0839 556610   Improve Libido Naturally

0839 556611   Beat Irritable Bowel Syndrome

0839 556612   Overcome Fatigue

0839 556613   Beat Migraine Naturally

0839 556614   Overcome Ovulation Pain

0839 556615   Directory

Index